Beyond Beautiful

Beyond Beautiful

A practical guide to being happy, confident,
and you in a looks-obsessed world

ANUSCHKA REES

ILLUSTRATIONS BY MARINA ESMERALDO

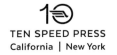

TEN SPEED PRESS
California | New York

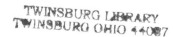

Contents

Part III Take back the power

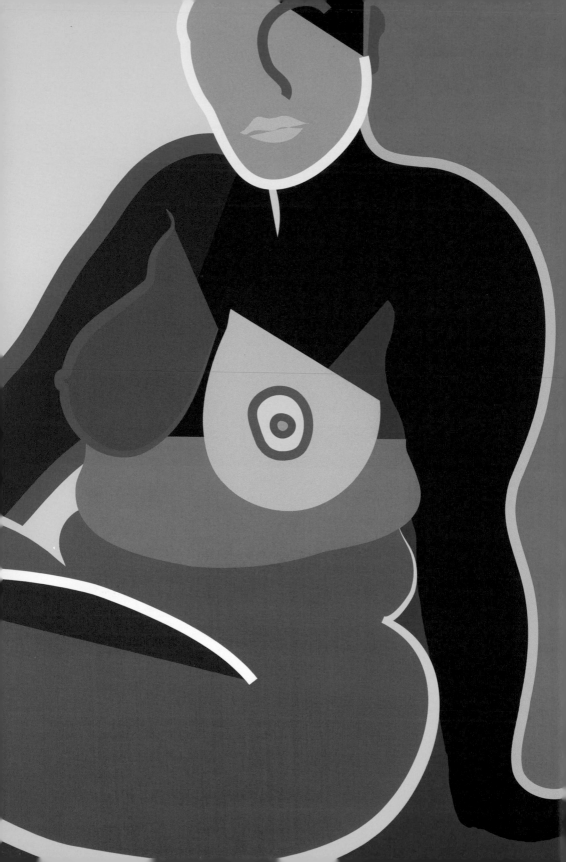

Introduction

Between flawless A-listers, ultralean fitness gurus, and picture-perfect social media celebrities, it's getting harder and harder to feel good about the way we look. Only one out of four women in the US likes her body. The cosmetic surgery industry is booming, with more than fifteen billion dollars spent yearly on procedures in the US alone. Two out of three women are on a diet at any given time, and even more shockingly, so are more than half of teenage girls.

It doesn't take a genius to figure out what's responsible for this epidemic of low body image among women and girls. We are bombarded with images of what we should look like from the moment we wake up: there's fitspiration, thinspiration, effortlessly chic fashion bloggers, and lingerie models in ad campaigns. Fit bodies, pretty faces, and perfect outfits are rewarded with attention and social media likes; imperfections like acne, "fashion fails," or extra pounds get ridiculed by commenters and gossip columnists.

The good news is that the beauty narrative in the media seems to be slowly shifting in a healthier direction. Body positivity has become a hot topic and, in response, plenty of brands have started using plus-size models in their campaigns or promised to stop retouching altogether. *Allure* magazine has banned the term "antiaging." Barbie no longer has a thigh gap and comes in a range of different body shapes. Progress!

But, of course, we're still quite a way from a perfectly diverse media landscape that doesn't teach girls and women to derive their self-worth from their appearance. And until then, we all desperately need a way to deal with the flood of picture-perfection on our screens.

One option: throw out your phone, TV, and computer. Or, you can read this book (wink, wink).

I stumbled upon the topic of body image after my first book, *The Curated Closet*, came out. The book is based on my own transformation from "die-hard shopaholic with a jam-packed wardrobe but nothing to wear" to "conscious consumer with a less-is-more attitude." I received lots of lovely messages from readers telling me how the steps in the book were working for them, and because the way we feel about our clothes is so tied to the way we feel about our looks, many of these women also told me about their body issues: about not feeling skinny, curvy, pretty, or young enough, and how social media has upped the pressure even more.

The more I thought and read about it, the more I understood the massive impact of body-image issues on women's lives. And I'm not even talking about the super serious stuff that low confidence is a risk factor for, like eating disorders, depression, or body dysmorphic disorder.

I mean all of the everyday things we do and feel because we were socialized to believe that our value is directly related to our appearance. Things like:

- Not being able to enjoy a night out with your friends because you're worried about how you look.

- Feeling stressed whenever someone with a camera approaches or having your day ruined by one bad photo that someone tagged you in.

- Dreading your next birthday because you're convinced it's all downhill from there.

- Pushing yourself to complete your beauty routine even when it feels like a chore.

- Feeling like your ability to find or keep love depends on your ability to stick to your diet.

- Not going after a work opportunity to speak in public because you feel too self-conscious.

- Feeling inhibited during sex.

- Trying one diet/beauty treatment/workout routine after another in the hopes of finally finding the magic bullet that's going to make you feel good about yourself.

- Declining an invitation to spend a day at the beach because you don't want people to see you in a bathing suit.

- Staying away from full-length mirrors to avoid being confronted with your body.

- Feeling like your weight is the main factor that's keeping you from being happy.

Imagine all the energy, time, and even money you would save if you suddenly felt fine about the way you look, and all the stuff you could do with it instead!

Of course, the fact that body image is a big problem is not a secret. Everyone from feminist bloggers to Hollywood actresses and even fashion magazines are talking about our society's unrealistic beauty ideals and the huge pressure that is put on women to fit that mold. But I noticed that there's one thing nobody talks about: a solution. Sure, we know how the media, fashion brands, and movie executives could improve the whole situation and, yes, it's important that we fix what's causing our insecurities at a systemic level. But does that mean that we're at the mercy of big brands and media outlets to finally stop promoting an unrealistic beauty standard? Is feeling insecure about our appearance just inevitable until further notice? Are we completely powerless?

"I'm intelligent, I'm a feminist, and I know that society's beauty ideal is BS. So why do I care so much about what I look like?"

I knew that couldn't be true. There are plenty of women who feel perfectly fine about their bodies, who aren't letting features that are commonly considered "flaws" get in the way of living their best lives. Also, if there is one thing I learned as a psychology grad student, it's that people's thoughts, feelings, and opinions are anything but set in stone. That's the entire basis of psychotherapy and self-development: you *can* change the way your mind works for the better, no matter the circumstances. That means you can also become more confident and stop seeing your body as some problem that needs fixing.

How? Well, that's what I still needed to find out. So I told my publisher that I wanted to write a practical book about body image, but I couldn't say exactly what I'd write about yet. All I knew were the questions I wanted this book to answer, such as:

- How am I ever supposed to feel good about myself when my culture is making it impossible?

- How can I stop feeling like an unhealthy slob whenever I scroll through my Instagram feed?

- How do I get over my fear of looking older?

- Should I get lip fillers to improve my confidence?

- How do I find the confidence to wear less makeup/ stop shaving/wear what I want?

My motivation was pretty strong because at almost thirty years old, I was still spending way too much time feeling like a self-conscious thirteen-year-old and even turning down work opportunities because I didn't feel "camera-ready." Fortunately, my publisher took a leap of faith, so I got to spend a year talking to some of the smartest people out there—psychologists, sociologists, media and women's studies experts, confidence coaches, and dieticians—and reading everything there is to read about body image, to see if I could find concrete, applicable advice for people (like me and pretty much every single woman I know) who feel like their insecurities are keeping them from living their best life. Spoiler alert: I found a ton of helpful and practical strategies that work and that go beyond wishy-washy calls to "love yourself" (uh . . . okay, but how exactly?).

Improving your body image isn't some weird hocus-pocus or brainwashing or lying to yourself. In fact, it's the opposite: it's about being *more* logical and seeing things more clearly than you have before.

Wanting to become more body-confident is also not a vain or trivial goal. Women's body image is a fundamentally feminist issue. According to Lexie Kite, body-image researcher and co-director of the nonprofit Beauty Redefined, "In a state of self-consciousness about our bodies, we perform worse on math tests and logical reasoning tests, our athletic performance goes down, and we have lower sexual assertiveness (including the ability to say 'no' when needed and discuss contraception)." Worrying about the way they look keeps girls from speaking up in class and women from going after leadership positions. It eats up time, energy, and mental capacity. Besides feeling shitty, a dent in your confidence can affect every area of your life—and improving your confidence has serious benefits that go far beyond simply liking what you see in the mirror. It can change your whole life.

Your body image includes not just how you feel about your actual neck-to-toe body, but also your thoughts about every other aspect of your appearance, and everything you do *because* of what you think about your looks, such as hiding behind your friends whenever a camera approaches, not raising a point in a team meeting because you don't want to attract attention to yourself, or spending hours at the gym because you've convinced you need to "tone up" to have fun this summer.

> "I often think that my life would be better if I were more attractive. Especially in summer, I see these girls with beautiful bodies who are comfortable running around in a bikini and tiny shorts. People seem to be drawn to them, and it just looks like they are having more fun."

It doesn't matter what exactly you don't like about your appearance for the tips and techniques that you'll find in this book to work. Body-image issues come in many different forms: some women worry about their weight, their skin, their body shape; some wish they had a smaller nose, fewer varicose veins, a narrower rib cage, a different skin tone, prettier feet, straighter teeth, smaller pores, no freckles, more freckles, a smaller butt, a bigger butt. But regardless of how small or all-encompassing your body worries are, or how trivial they may seem to someone else, they are not something you have to live with.

#beyondbeautiful

For more resources, tools, advice, and personal stories, or to share your own story: Visit the BB community on Instagram (@beyondbeautifulbook) or at beyondbeautifulbook.com.

How to get the most out of this book

There is a big difference between understanding something on a conscious level and actually internalizing it. That is why it's important that you don't just read this book, but really work with it. There are two types of exercises in this book.

Reflection questions

Don't skip these! And for maximum effect, complete them in writing. Find a nice empty notebook and challenge yourself to dig deep and be totally honest with yourself: nobody will see these answers but you.

The Beyond Beautiful toolbox

This is an arsenal of practical techniques that you can use over and over again to deal with anything the body-image gods may throw at you, from a callous lover's body-shaming comment to a surprise pool party with cameras everywhere.

Improving your body image is a process, so don't make this a weekend project. If you rush the exercises, any new perspectives you gain won't have enough time to permeate and stick. Take it chapter by chapter and always give yourself the time you need to reflect on what you just read and perhaps even discuss the exercises with a friend.

When to seek professional help

Sometimes self-help is not enough. Because sometimes, feeling down about the way you look can also be a symptom of something more serious, such as an eating disorder, depression, or body dysmorphic disorder, which causes people to have a distorted view of their body and obsess over nonexistent or minor flaws for hours a day.

According to Roberto Olivardia, clinical psychologist and lecturer at the Harvard Medical School, a key sign that someone may be in the middle of a clinical body-image disorder is that they are willing to go to extreme lengths to fix their self-perceived flaw: "Compulsive exercise, restricting foods, use of laxatives, diet pills, anabolic steroid use, [and] binge eating and purging are just some of the things people do when they are in a dangerous territory regarding their bodies." Even if you do none of these things, it's important to reach out for help if your body-image worries feel overwhelming, consume a large chunk of your thoughts, or make you feel worthless or unlovable.

A good first step is talking to your doctor, who will then refer you to a specialist. You can also ask your insurance company for a list of doctors and therapists who specialize in treating body-image issues, and call directly to make an appointment. If you don't have insurance, many community health centers also provide counseling and mental health care for free or at a low cost. You can find your local health center here: https://findahealthcenter.hrsa.gov.

For immediate emotional support, advice, and information, call the free 24/7 crisis hotline at 1-800-273-8255.

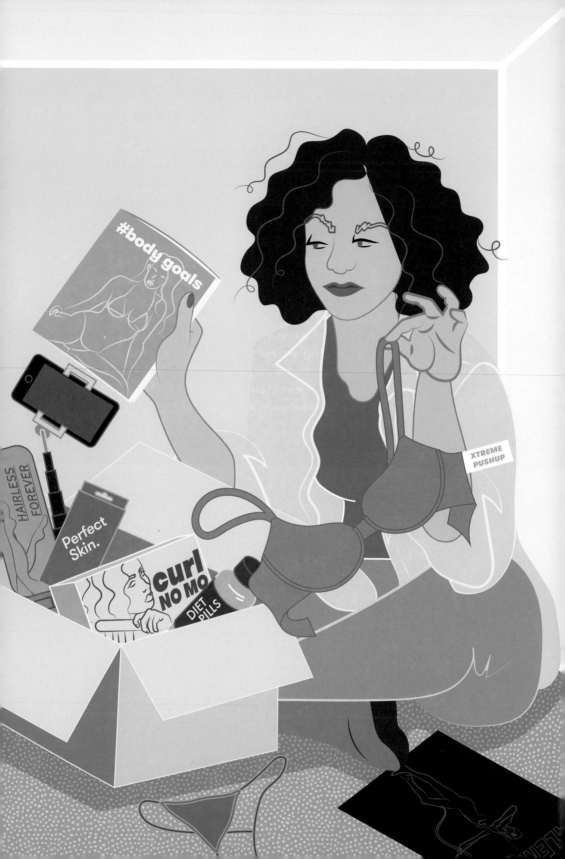

PART I

UNPACK THE PROBLEM

CHAPTER 1

BODY IMAGE 101

A healthy body image is a bit like a great work-life balance: we know we definitely want it, but we're also not 100 percent clear on what it actually looks like, or how to get it. And the fact that body image is a hot topic right now hasn't made things any more straightforward; because mixed in with all of the good advice, there is a whole bunch of conflicting information and misconceptions that have muddied the waters even further.

Is it more empowering to work hard in the gym to get the body I want, or to accept my body as it is? Should I get a boob job/Botox/lip injections to feel more comfortable in my skin, or would that mean succumbing to sexist beauty ideals? Does wanting bigger boobs make me a bad feminist? Should I even be thinking so much about my body image, or is that just adding to my fixation over how my body looks?

Questions after questions.

So before we get practical, let's clear this up once and for all. What exactly is this thing we call "a healthy body image"?

Self-esteem, confidence, body image: What's the difference?

When it comes to body image, a lot of different terms get thrown around. So to make sure we're all on the same page, here is a quick overview of the key concepts.

Self-esteem

Your self-esteem is your general opinion about your worth
as a person. It is a product of all of the messages you have
internalized about yourself and—crucially—the various
groups you belong to (like Americans, art majors, extroverts,
and so on). Someone with a healthy self-esteem knows
they have flaws just like everyone else, but they generally
think of themselves as a good person who is worthy of
being loved, respected, and treated well. People with an
unhealthy self-esteem believe that they are somehow infe-
rior to others. They are very critical of themselves and tend
to focus mainly on their mistakes and weaknesses; at the
same time, they ignore or downplay positive experiences
like compliments or achievements. Some people's negative
self-esteem is so ingrained that it affects everything they
do. For others, self-esteem issues only pop up in especially
difficult, stressful situations.

Confidence

In contrast to self-esteem, confidence has little to do with
how much you value yourself, but rather with how much
you believe you can *do* things well, whether that is achiev-
ing your career goals, holding your own in a conversation,
or keeping a houseplant alive. Confidence is often very
specific and most always earned: You feel confident in
your spelling because you have been practicing since
preschool, and you feel confident about not getting lost
in a foreign city because you have been on similar vacations before. Conversely, you may not feel confident in
your spelling when learning a foreign language, and if
you have never been abroad, you may feel much more
nervous in a new city because you haven't racked up any
confidence points for that specific situation yet. In the best-
case scenario, your confidence for specific things turns
into global confidence, where you feel like you can learn
or figure out most things if you try. Stanford psychologist
Carol Dweck calls this the "growth mind-set."

Body image

Your body image is the portion of your overall self-esteem that relates to your appearance. Just like the rest of your self-esteem, your body image is based on all of the messages you have picked up about your appearance from early childhood on, as well as messages about your "type" of look, such as blondes, people with acne, pear-shaped bodies, and so on. Psychologists believe that body image makes up an average of one-third of a person's self-esteem. But that figure can vary considerably. For some people, what they look like has almost zero significance to them. For others, how they feel about their appearance (whether that's good or bad) has a huge influence on their self-worth.

"So . . . how I feel about my looks has nothing to do with confidence?"

Correct. Although "confidence" or "(not) feeling confident" are perhaps the most common terms people use to talk about how they feel about their body, *technically* whether we do or don't like our appearance is not a matter of confidence, but of self-esteem (and specifically body image). But, since there really isn't a smooth way to say "has a healthy body image" or "has a healthy self-esteem," for the sake of all of us I will continue using the term "confident" throughout the book in the way that it is commonly understood.

> **"Self-esteem isn't everything; it's just that there's nothing without it."**
>
> Gloria Steinem

Five myths about body image you probably believe

Now that you're up to speed on the terminology, it's time we start busting some of the peskiest myths about body image that are currently floating about in our media sphere.

MYTH 1 Body confidence equals thinking you look good

No other myth is a clearer reflection of our society's looks-obsession than this one. How could you possibly have a healthy relationship with your body unless you thought it looked attractive? If you had a healthy body image, you, too, would be spending all day taking nude selfies, showing off your bod in teeny bikinis, and feeling great all around, like all those ultraconfident, body-loving influencers and fearless, flawless pop stars. Right?

Nope. Thinking you're hot stuff is not the pinnacle of body confidence. And to build a better body image you do not need to somehow convince yourself of your aesthetic appeal. What you do need to do is fix your buggy self-worth barometer and understand that your physical appearance (whether you fit the current beauty ideal or not) is just a single, volatile, and not even particularly interesting aspect of yourself. You are worthy for a whole set of other reasons.

"WHAT'S THE POINT, THEN? I JUST WANT TO FEEL BEAUUUTIFUL!"

If you are now thinking something along these lines, ask yourself *why* you want beauty. I don't need to have met you in person to know that you don't have an intrinsic desire to achieve physical perfection for its own sake, but that you want what everyone wants: to feel worthy, happy, loved. And just like every other woman out there, you have been taught that being attractive is your best chance of getting there. Of course, it's exactly this toxic belief that fuels body-image issues in the first place, causing you to feel, well . . . less worthy, less happy, and less loved.

Having a healthy body image doesn't mean resigning yourself to a mirrorless life wearing nothing but potato sacks. The goal here is not to convince you to stop brushing your hair and swear off makeup, bikini waxes, and glute exercises forever. All you are trying to do is to simply turn down the power beauty ideals hold over you by a notch or three. And once you have done the work, you may well end up liking what you see in the mirror more than you used to. But in the grand scheme of things, that will only be a pleasant side effect.

MYTH 2 You need to "fix" your appearance to fix your confidence

Ever since body positivity and female empowerment have become major topics in mainstream culture, we've developed a zero-tolerance policy toward sexist ads, discriminatory casting, and anything else that suggests women need to look a certain way to be considered attractive. Ironically, we're still totally fine with brands, magazines, and influencers encouraging us to improve our appearance—as long as it's in the name of confidence and self-care.

Do you feel self-conscious in a bikini? This 12-week work-out and diet plan is going to help you love yourself again! You're worried about the lines on your forehead? Treat yourself to a paycheck's worth of skin-care products and a pinch of Botox! You don't like your face? Let me show you these empowering makeup tricks to make it look so much better. You're unhappy with your post-baby body? If invasive surgery is what it takes for you to feel good in your skin, then you owe it to yourself.

And in theory, all of this makes sense: when something is making you feel self-conscious, then changing it should make you more confident, right? Sure, but that something is never your body. You don't feel self-conscious or insecure or unhappy because of the way your thighs, your face, or your boobs look. You're unhappy because of the millions of messages that have drilled into you that your thighs, face, or boobs could even have an effect on your happiness to begin with.

So instead of further advertising beauty as a magic bullet and looking better as the only path to confidence, we need to start sending and receiving the message that confidence is an inside job. Instead of encouraging women to spend even more time, energy, and money on their appearance, we need to help them feel worthy and happy in a bikini, without makeup, or post-pregnancy—regardless of how much they happen to fit the current beauty ideal. Because the road to confidence is not fixing your appearance—it's fixing your mind-set.

MYTH 3 Improving your body image is about learning to L-O-V-E your body

Self-love has become a bit of a buzzword lately, and many a conversation on body image ends on the note, "Just love your body, that's the most important thing." Now, if you already feel like you love your body, then kudos to you, you're ahead of the curve. But as a strategy, when you're riding the body-image struggle bus, "just love your body" is pretty useless. First, it's terribly unclear advice. How am I supposed to spontaneously conjure up warm feelings for my body parts? Is there a button I can push to make that happen? Second, the idea that loving your body is a prerequisite to feeling happy and secure can add a huge amount of—totally unnecessary—pressure.

People with a healthy body image don't love their hips or their waist any more than their lungs or their sense of balance. Looking in the mirror doesn't give them a tingly jolt of happy energy. In fact, the reason they're at peace with their bodies is precisely because they *don't* have strong feelings about their physical appearances. How they look is only one of many factors they use to establish how they feel about themselves.

Obviously, the advice to love your body comes from a well-meaning place. But it's also misleading because it keeps women stuck on their mirror image by reinforcing the idea that their physical form is the gatekeeper to happiness. Yes, you should strive to cultivate respect and compassion for yourself, as a human being, and your body (including the way it looks) is a part of that. But if your goal is to be happy and feel confident, understanding that *you are more than your body* is miles more valuable than writing love letters to your individual body parts.

MYTH 4 People with a healthy body image don't care what others think of their looks

While I was researching this book I noticed that many women seem to think of body confidence as nice-in-theory but essentially unattainable, because they believe it would require them to turn into some fearless Samantha Jones—type character who gives zero fucks about anyone's opinion of her. "It took me a week to recover when my colleague pointed out the zit on my chin, and you expect me to just not care at all what people think about me?"

Actually, no. Humans are social creatures. All of us, no matter how great our body image, care about how we appear to others. We want them to think all the good stuff about us: that we're smart, compassionate, successful, trustworthy, fun to be around, and pleasant-looking is on that list, too. Even people with a healthy body image may get a boost from a compliment, ask for a second opinion for the haircut they are considering, or spend extra time doing their makeup for a date.

And just like everyone else, people with a healthy body image may feel a little down when someone makes an off-hand comment about the way they look. But the difference is that it doesn't ruin their day or affect their decisions in a major way, because "looking good" is, if at all, just one of many qualities they base their self-worth on.

"CONFIDENT PEOPLE WOULD NEVER GO ON A DIET"

Related to the myth that being confident equals being immune to outside opinions is this idea that someone truly confident would also never want to change anything about their appearance. And that going on a diet, getting cosmetic surgery, or wearing a weave is proof of someone's shaky relationship with their body. In some online circles, celebrities who are "caught" trying to lose weight on purpose after showing allegiance to body positivity are essentially considered traitors. If they really believed in the cause, if they really "loved themselves," they would also love their body as it is.

In any other area of our lives, that same logic would be considered ridiculous. You have probably made it a goal to change something about yourself before. Perhaps you wanted to stop procrastinating, or go to bed earlier, or stop snapping at people when you are stressed. But does that mean you didn't have respect for yourself or judge other procrastinators or night owls? Of course not! When you have a healthy body image, you understand that your appearance is just one small aspect of yourself. And if something about that small aspect is not serving you well, you may make the executive decision to change it—no biggie.

MYTH 5 You're a bad feminist if you don't like the way you look

While it's important that we recognize body image as a feminist issue, that F-label can cause quite a bit of cognitive dissonance when you consider yourself a feminist, but your own body wish list aligns with the sexist societal norms you so reject. "I hate how women are objectified, I hate our toxic diet culture, the 'skinny is better' ideal, all of that. So why do I get so excited when my jeans fit a little looser than normal? Why do I catch myself envying my well-endowed friends? Am I actually much less woke than I thought I was?"

Besides making you question the steadfastness of your beliefs, all of that internal conflict—all of that feeling bad about feeling bad about yourself—may tempt you to just ignore or downplay your insecurities instead of facing them head-on. Alternatively, you may reframe your collective ideals as purely individual ones: "I *personally* just feel so much better sans fuzz on my legs, which has nothing to do with societal norms, thank you very much!"

But cultural socialization is a powerful thing. On an intellectual level, you may not *want* to like slim bodies, large breasts, petite noses, or hair-free legs, but when you grow up surrounded by messages telling you those things equal beauty, then honestly it would be very impressive if you hadn't internalized those ideals to at least some degree.

And that's okay, because when it comes to your identity as a feminist, what you like or don't like is kind of beside

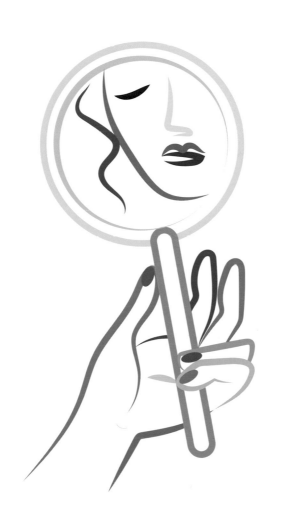

the point. Can you only qualify as vegetarian if you hate the taste of meat? No! It's your personal convictions and choices that make you a vegetarian—whether you like bacon and pepperoni pizza is irrelevant. And what makes you a feminist is not the extent to which your personal aesthetic preferences align with society's beauty ideals, but the fact that you a) understand that these ideals are discriminatory and harmful and b) are doing your bit to fight them.

The vicious cycle of feeling not-so-great about the way you look

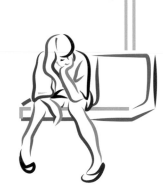

According to psychologist Joel Kevin Thompson, body image consists of three components: the mental picture you have of the way you look, your emotions and thoughts about that picture, and your actions in response to it (anything you do to improve or maintain your appearance; for example, dieting or wearing makeup).

A key point to remember is that these components all reinforce each other.

On one hand, that's a bummer because it means that it's very easy to get stuck in a negative cycle where you feel bad about your body and your actions (such as efforts to fix or cover up your "flaws") push you even further down your shame spiral. But on the other hand, it also means that if you can manage to move just one of the three factors in a more positive direction—your mental image of your body, your interpretation of that image, or your behavior—the other two will follow.

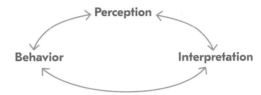

In this book, we'll tackle your bad body image from all three angles: we'll fix your likely very wonky self-perception, we'll change how you feel and think about what you see in the mirror, and we'll make sure that your actions when it comes to everything from social media to food, fitness, style, and beauty help you take back the power, instead of contributing to your confidence funk.

So prepare to get stuck in a new cycle, but this time, a happy, body-confident one!

Avoiding and chasing: The two ways we deal with body-image stress

You probably know exactly how your body image is making you feel: self-conscious, inadequate, stressed out, envious, perhaps even a little angry. But what you may not be aware of is the extent to which your body image is also affecting your actions. All the things you do and don't do to cope with feeling not quite (or at all) "good enough." There are two coping strategies you may be using to some degree at the moment: avoiding and chasing.

COPING STRATEGY 1: Avoiding

Avoiding—the head-in-the-sand way of dealing with body-image stress—comes in two major forms: hiding and running. Whenever you are trying to camouflage the parts of your appearance that you feel insecure about, you are using the first type: hiding. The obvious tools most people use for this strategy are makeup and clothes, of course, but there are plenty of other ways to hide: for example by posing a certain way to cover your "bad side," holding your hand over a "flaw" whenever you meet people, or having a friend stand in front of you in photos.

"It will be well over 100 degrees outside this year in the summer, and I'll be in jeans and a long-sleeved shirt. I haven't worn shorts since I was eleven, because I think my legs are too thick."

The second type of avoiding, running, is what you do when you avoid situations that could expose or highlight the parts of yourself that you feel self-conscious about. Here are some common situations people may run from:

- The beach, the pool, and other places that call for swimwear or otherwise revealing types of clothes

- Exercising or dancing in public

- Places or events where you might be photographed or videotaped

- Parties and other events where you feel you would need to wear clothes that draw attention to your "flaws" or simply draw attention to you at all

- Situations where your hair or makeup may get messed up or where you couldn't wear any

- Places where others may see you (partially) undressed, such as the doctor's office, gym locker rooms, or spas

- Places with lots of mirrors, such as changing rooms in stores, hairdressers, or gyms

- Places with a potentially high density of attractive or fashionable people

- Seeing people who may comment on the way you look (such as friends or relatives)

The logic behind avoidance behaviors is simple: if others can't see my flaws, they won't judge me for them. But it's important to note that just as often people run or hide not because they are worried about what others think, but to avoid having to confront the way they look *themselves*. This is often why people hate having their photo taken. They're afraid others will see it, but they're even *more* afraid of the emotional pain they know they would experience if they saw the bad photo themselves.

"I barely ever go to bars or clubs. All the other girls seem to look almost perfect, and I have just no idea what to do to look better or at least feel better about how I look."

WHY AVOIDING HURTS YOUR BODY IMAGE

Not only does not being able to do what you want to do and imposing strict rules on yourself feel shitty, but it also reinforces your insecurities.

Remember the negative body-image cycle from page 23? Our thoughts, emotions, and actions all affect each other. Every time you wear baggy clothes to hide your thighs or stay on your towel while your friends have fun swimming in the ocean, you are telling your subconscious that your insecurities are valid. By letting go of your avoidance habit, you stop feeding that flame and, equally valuable, you are also giving yourself the opportunity to notice that nothing bad actually happens when you expose your flaws. People treat you the same way; nobody cares. That realization alone can often work wonders and help you overcome or at least tone down the shame you have attached to your flaws.

"I can't go to the beach because I keep thinking I'll look like a little ten-year-old boy running around with a bulging belly."

COPING STRATEGY 2: Chasing

Instead of covering up their flaws and staying away from activities that would expose them, some people respond to feelings of inadequacy in a very different way: by tightening the reins to control the situation and chasing beauty ideals. Classic moves include:

- Dedicating big chunks of free time to improving or maintaining your appearance

- Following a strict and elaborate beauty routine

- Perpetual dieting

- Closely monitoring your looks by taking regular mirror pics or measurements, or weighing yourself daily, followed by overanalyzing that data

- Adhering to your own extreme grooming standards (such as never leaving the house without perfect brows or freshly shaven legs)

- Constantly researching new beauty products that will help fix a perceived flaw

- Going to extreme measures to protect your looks or prevent aging, such as completely avoiding the sun

- Responding to body-image blows (such as an offhand comment or a bad photo) with an even more elaborate beauty routine

- Considering a laundry list of cosmetic treatments, including plastic surgery

Chasers have the motivation to do this type of stuff because it gives them a feeling of accomplishment. And why wouldn't it? If you believe your ability to be happy depends on your appearance, any type of beauty treatment will make you feel proactive, hopeful, and even like you are making a smart investment in your future—just like putting a fat chunk of cash in your savings account gives you a sense of gratification because it makes you feel like a smart, accomplished grown-up.

Of course, the reverse is also true: things that *reduce* your attractiveness seem like a huge threat to your livelihood. This is why people with a shaky body image—even when they are happy with the way they look—will often spend considerable energy on their appearance to maintain it—for example, by closely monitoring their weight, tracking their food, and doing everything in their power to prevent aging.

"I have a very extensive skin-care routine. I haven't decided if I started it for the self-care aspect, or because I'm scared of aging and 'losing' my youth and beauty. Probably both . . . "

WHY CHASING HURTS YOUR BODY IMAGE

There are plenty of reasons *chasing* is no good, all of which we will talk about in detail later on. For now, let's focus on the two biggies. First, a chaser's routine costs a huge amount of time, energy, and money. Second, chasing reinforces the single most toxic belief that lies at the heart of body-image troubles: that your happiness and worth depend on your looks. Because after investing all of that energy into your appearance, you're much more likely to attribute positive experiences, whether that's a friendly interaction or praise at work, to your improved appearance.

This feedback loop is a key reason why women and men with a tendency to chase will often develop more and more intense beauty routines for themselves and why so many of those who opt for cosmetic surgery once come back for more. They believe their looks play a crucial role in any of the good stuff that happens to them, so naturally the path to even *more* happiness must be to look even better.

"I know I have a good body, but it's hard work and sometimes I wish I could just take a break from working out and being so careful about what I eat."

When do you hide, run, or chase?

Most people with body insecurities will use both coping strategies—avoiding and chasing—at different times, often depending on the context. For example, you may not allow yourself to wear short sleeves because of your "fat" upper arms, but also be looking into "fixing" your lips with injections. You may at some point turn down an invitation to a party, but a couple of months later respond to a similar invitation by drafting an intense workout routine in preparation and vow to look your best by the time the party rolls around.

"I hate the cellulite on my thighs and have spent so much money trying to get rid of it, from dry-brushing to expensive lotions to radio-frequency therapy. Nothing has worked, and I can't believe I will have to spend another summer sweating in long pants."

Do you have a go-to coping strategy? Do you use one or the other for different situations? Think about a typical day in your life, and list everything you do to **hide, run,** or **chase** on a regular basis.

Which of these actions feel the most burdensome to you? Which do you wish you didn't have to do most often?

You're not the boss of me

The fact that coping strategies reinforce a less-than-ideal body image is not the only reason you should work towards letting go of them. It's also about reclaiming control over your life.

When you're using a lot of coping strategies on a daily basis (whether consciously or subconsciously), your insecurities are making decisions for you and running the show. Your judgy inner voice is keeping you on a tight leash, telling you to never let anyone see your "flaws," to never miss a step in your strict beauty routine, and to do everything in your power to look better.

Letting go of coping habits means having the freedom to spend your life outside of these constraints. The freedom to accept invitations and opportunities, even if bikinis and high-def cameras are involved; to wear makeup when you feel like it, not because you'd be self-conscious without it; to choose workouts based on how much fun they are rather than how many calories they burn; to wear clothes because you like them, not because they flatter your figure or cover up "flaws"; and to simply enjoy life without worrying about what you look like.

What is your biggest insecurity when it comes to your appearance?

"Definitely my weight. I cannot even count how many times I've lost and regained the same twenty pounds. When I'm in my skinny phase I feel confident and happy (though hungry and most likely cranky because of that). When I am on the fatter end of my spectrum I feel like I haven't got it together, like I am letting myself down."

"I have fine hair all over my body, including my butt and back, and I am VERY self-conscious about this. I will not wear any shirt that shows my back or even dips too low on the back of my neck."

"My biggest insecurity is the color of my skin. Americans find this hard to understand, but I am Indian and have actually been told things like I have sinned in a past life and as punishment, I was born dark-skinned. People have said to my parents, 'Good luck getting your daughter married!' and my own grandma slathers me in 'whitening' creams to try to get me to be whiter."

"The list of things I'm self-conscious about could fill a book: all the weight I carry on my torso, my lack of a butt, my collarbone and shoulders which are sort of sloping and rounded, my square face, my double chin, my fine hair, my untoned biceps, having too-big breasts, my cellulite, etc., etc., etc."

"Body image is so weird as a queer person. I've even been thinking quite a bit about getting a radical breast reduction because having this feminine chest makes me so uncomfortable in a way that I feel like only other queer people understand."

"I'm happy to say that I like most parts of my body, but my thighs annoy me from a practical point of view when they painfully rub against each other when I'm sweating. Wearing biker shorts underneath skirts in warm climates solves this, though."

"I hate my large breasts. They've led me to be overly sexualized my entire life, and it's difficult to dress them."

"My worst nightmare is being forced to wear a bikini because I have this fear of anybody seeing my stomach. Sometimes I dream about having surgery to just slice it off and I fantasize about what it must be like to have a flat stomach."

"My biggest insecurity is getting older and therefore wrinklier and saggier."

"As a teenager I felt a lot of shame about the parts of my body most visibly affected by my cerebral palsy. Slowly, with the help of my friends, my family, and the online disability community, I am learning to think of those parts not as 'broken' but simply as 'different' but no less worthy."

**BEYOND
BEAUTIFUL
TOOLBOX**

Say hi to your judgy inner voice

One of the most important milestones on the path to a better body image is realizing that, really, it's not you—it's *them*. Your insecurities aren't a natural consequence of your appearance, and they are definitely not an integral part of who you are. All of those negative thoughts you have about your body have a clear external source. It's not really you talking, it's your judgy inner voice—the product of years of socialization.

Some people like to refer to this voice as their inner critic, but personally, I think that gives it a little too much credit. Your judgy inner voice isn't critically examining all the facts before it tells you that you look ridiculous wearing a miniskirt, that you need to go on a diet, or that your life would be better if your nose were smaller, your boobs bigger, and your skin clearer—it's simply spouting off it's little superficial mantras any chance it gets. I like to think of my negative inner voice as a tiny, Grumpy-Cat—faced gremlin that sits in my ear and considers it its job to periodically remind me of all of my physical flaws throughout the day. Author Melissa Ambrosini calls this her inner mean girl, which works perfectly, too.

Throughout this book, you'll come across lots of practical techniques for dealing with your very own judgy inner voice. But for now, just say hi and get to know each other!

Step 1

Is your judgy inner voice a classic bully à la *Mean Girls'* Regina George, a gremlin, or perhaps a middle-aged white guy in a suit? Picture exactly what it looks like, how it talks, how it moves. And give it a name, too! I've named mine Calvin.

From now on, make a point of picturing your gremlin/mean girl whenever negative thoughts about your appearance pop into your head.

Step 2

For three days, track everything your judgy inner voice throws at you. Write down these three pieces of information:

- The trigger that made your voice speak up. For example: seeing yourself in a photo, your pants feeling a little tight, scrolling through Instagram, walking into the gym, a comment someone made, and so on.

- The exact phrase it used. For example: "You look enormous" or "If you were prettier, you'd already have your drink."

- Your response, whether it's a specific action (like canceling an invitation or going on a diet) or an emotion (anger, shame, sadness, guilt, and so on).

Feel free to also add other common things your inner voice says that didn't come up during your three days of tracking. For example, if you tend to feel insecure when shopping for clothes or going swimming, add that to your list, too.

Step 3

After three days of tracking, look over your list and identify:

- Your key triggers (specific situations, people, and so on)

- Your biggest pain points (which of the many things your inner voice throws at you tend to hit the hardest? Comments about your weight or your skin? Hints that your boyfriend may lose interest or strangers could be judging you?)

- Your go-to response (are you most likely to feel sad, embarrassed, angry? Do you respond to insecurities by removing yourself from the situation or by trying harder to conform to beauty ideals?)

Step 4

Now that you've identified your judgy inner voice's spiel, you have all the intel you need to prepare a few punchy comebacks. To help you out in the future, these comebacks should be more than simple "You suck, fuck beauty standards" assertions, but make innate sense to you and describe exactly what your judgy inner voice is getting wrong. If you struggle to come up with much right now, don't worry. As you work through this book, you'll pick up plenty of ammunition that you can use to talk back to your judgy inner voice and stop it from having the last word ever again.

TRIGGER I caught my reflection in a shop window.

INNER VOICE SAYS "Wow, your thighs look like tree trunks. You should not be wearing shorts."

ORIGINAL RESPONSE Felt uncomfortable for the rest of the day.

HOW I'LL TALK BACK NEXT TIME "It's not my job to look as skinny as possible, I have better things to do, and I deserve to feel cool and comfortable like everyone else."

TRIGGER Someone tagged me in a photo from last week's party.

INNER VOICE SAYS "How embarrassing that you were having fun all night while your skin looked this horrible and everyone could see."

ORIGINAL RESPONSE Untagged myself from all photos of that night and vowed to stay in when my acne looks extra bad.

HOW I'LL TALK BACK NEXT TIME "I am not going to allow unrealistic beauty ideals to restrict my freedom and keep me from living life to the fullest. I was having a great time that night and the fact that I happened to have a hormonal acne-flare up at the same time does not take anything away from that."

TRIGGER While waiting for my friend at a bar I overheard two guys talking about how amazing another girl's butt looks.

INNER VOICE SAYS "If you didn't have such a saggy, flat butt, they would be talking to you right now and you wouldn't have to sit here all lonely."

ORIGINAL RESPONSE Had two extra glasses of wine and spent the subway ride home staring at Instagram models with perfect behinds.

HOW I'LL TALK BACK NEXT TIME "I am intelligent, compassionate and headed for big things. If a single piece of my anatomy really keeps someone from wanting to get to know me, then I've dodged one hell of a bullet."

CHAPTER 2

THE MEDIA

Never before has there been so much media buzz and public support for female empowerment and diversity issues. We no longer live in the '60s when no one would bat an eye over body-shaming ad slogans like "A wife can blame herself if she loses love by getting middle-age skin," or "[A pear] is no shape for a girl."

Today we have body-positivity campaigns, feminist hashtags, and plus-size supermodels. We applaud authenticity. Fitness bloggers and celebrities show off "flaws" like cellulite, acne, or stretch marks on social media to make the point that all of that stuff is natural and nothing to be ashamed about. Brands, magazines, and film studios face immediate backlash for obvious photoshopping, nondiverse casting, and anything else that could potentially reinforce unrealistic beauty standards or gender stereotypes. And yet, despite all of the empowering messages we see in the media, women today are no less self-conscious about their appearance than they've always been. Why?

The beauty blast

Perhaps the most basic reason why women worldwide still feel so much pressure when it comes to their appearance is that we are simply more exposed to beauty in the digital age. Beauty ideals have always existed, but while our grandmothers saw images of our society's beauty ideal perhaps just a few times a day, on TV or in magazines, we are confronted with them all day, every day. From the time we check our phone in the morning to the moment we hit the couch for a bit of late-night TV, our screens reliably feed us a steady diet of female bodily perfection, supplemented, of course, by old-school beauty dispensaries like magazines and billboards.

Our beauty-heavy daily routine has two major consequences. First, we internalize the media's narrow and
unrealistic beauty ideals and eventually start judging our
own appearance through the same impossible lens. If every
single woman who represents beauty in the media, be it in
ads, in magazines, or in movies, is young, slim, and light-
skinned, there's simply no way you can't *not* start thinking of
those qualities as the gold standard.

Second, we learn that beauty matters . . . big time. When
we watch TV shows or scroll through our feeds, we don't
just *see* beautiful people, we also witness how others talk
about them and how they get better opportunities. We
hear how people celebrate and admire beauty as if it is a
major achievement. We watch women who fit our culture's beauty ideals being fawned over in movies, on red
carpets, and on talk shows. We notice that all the leading
ladies in Hollywood movies are gorgeous, the prettiest
Instagrammers have the biggest followings, and songs are
only ever about the beautiful ones, not the okay-looking
ones with a great sense of humor.

At the same time, we also see what happens to women
who don't fit into our society's idea of beauty. We see how
celebrities are scrutinized, even ridiculed, in tabloid magazines, on talk shows, and on online message boards for
having cellulite or armpit hair, for having gained weight, or
for trying something new with their clothes. All of this tells
us that as women in this world, the way we look influences
everything: success, love, and how well people treat us.

**"There's a reason that Elizabeth Bennett's looks are
mentioned before her great wit, her voracious appetite
for reading, and her overall intellect. Looks sell books."**

The real cause of low body confidence

Most people believe that the unrealistic beauty ideal we are bombarded with is what's solely responsible for women's low body confidence. But actually, that is only the tip of the iceberg. Considering yourself (or parts of yourself) unattractive does not automatically lead to a bad body image. For those beauty ideals to affect you, you also need to believe that your own attractiveness is even relevant to begin with. You need to be convinced that it has an impact on your happiness.

You probably know plenty of people who are fully aware they are never going to win a beauty contest, and yet they are not afraid to wear swimwear in public, be photographed, or speak in front of an audience. Their body image is fine, because they simply don't believe that their happiness depends on their looks. On the other hand, you probably also know people who do happen to fit our culture's beauty ideals and still find plenty of faults intheir appearance, people who anyone would put in the "good-looking" category but who nevertheless feel very insecure about their appearance.

I bet you know way more women than men who fit that second group. Because when you live in a world that teaches you that your value depends on your appearance, every tiny weight gain, every stretch mark, and every expression line is a real threat. Ten extra pounds means the difference between having fun at a party and feeling self-conscious all night. A little razor burn on your bikini line means the difference between feeling sexy and wanting to turn off the lights to make sure your partner won't get grossed out. A zit on your cheek means the difference between kicking ass in a meeting and not speaking up because you don't want to attract attention to yourself.

The belief that beauty matters is what's causing women to be so deathly afraid of showing signs of aging, to attribute achievements and positive interactions to their looks instead of their spirit, and to consider a five-thousand-dollar boob job the smartest investment they could make in their future happiness. Yes, our narrow beauty ideals are a huge problem, and we'll talk plenty about how to deal with them in this book. And, yes, it is a step forward that we are now seeing more diversity in the media, and it's important that we keep promoting that cause. But we also have to start tackling the root of the whole problem: that beauty matters so damn much in the first place.

Why "I'm just doing this for myself" is BS

Interestingly, a lot of women don't realize how much the portrayal of beauty in the media affects them. In a study conducted by Dove in 2010, 72 percent of women said they feel a huge amount of pressure to look attractive. However, the majority of those women believed that any pressure they felt, they put on themselves—only 17 percent admitted to feeling pressured by society.

But let's get something straight: just because it's your hand that's reaching for the razor every morning does not mean society had nothing to do with it. Just because no one is holding a knife to your throat to force you to drop that cookie or call up the beauty doc does not mean you are making these choices from a place of freedom. Sure, you are free to stop wearing makeup, to stop shaving, to stop wearing bras, to stop dieting, to stop doing everything in your power to look attractive. But what you, as a woman, are not free to do is to stop any of these things without incurring the consequences: scrutiny, comments, fewer opportunities, and even outright body-shaming.

Feeling "uncomfortable" when you've gained weight, aren't wearing makeup, or didn't shave is a consequence, too, but it's only an indirect one. If you were stranded alone on a desert island, do you think you would care one bit about your belly pooch, side profile, or hairy legs? No. If you hadn't grown up in this culture, you would have never even had the idea that something as inherently natural as leg hair could ever be a detriment to your well-being.

Of course, no one wants to be a puppet without free will. Admitting that "I feel really bad about my body . . ." or "I spend a ton of time and effort on my appearance . . ." or "I am getting this nose job or liposuction or breast lift . . . because I've learned that beauty matters in this society" clashes with our entire value system. But if we want to reduce the pull that our society's beauty narrative has on our daily life, it's crucial that we acknowledge that the ideals we are judging ourselves by are not our own. Because only then can we start distancing ourselves from them.

Pretty little things

As if blasting us with beauty weren't already enough, the media also shapes our body image in another, much more insidious way: by teaching us a certain perspective of thinking of women's bodies. From makeover shows to "Who wore it better?" to beauty pageants, red carpet photo calls, and "Hot 100" lists, a large chunk of mainstream media centers around admiring and ranking women's appearances. And that's a problem.

"If you are a woman, people will see your looks first. When male politicians go on the podium, they are judged by their presentation and words. When female politicians stand up, every journalist writes about their outfits!"

When the predominant way the female body is presented in the media is as an *object* whose main purpose is to be evaluated, then we ourselves (whether we are male or female) can't help but use that same perspective to judge the female bodies we see in real life, including our own. Studies have shown over and over again how being exposed to objectifying images and media messages leads to *self-objectifying*. Girls and women start thinking of their own bodies primarily as something to be looked at and desired by *others*. A good body is a body that *others* find beautiful and sexy.

To a certain degree, it's normal to think about and try to manage what others may see when they look at you. But self-objectifying becomes a problem when you are habitually paying more attention to how you may be perceived rather than how you are perceiving others and what you are experiencing. One woman in my survey said this about her self-monitoring habits: "I'm so constantly aware of my body/face/outfit that I sometimes feel like I'm looking at myself in the third person. In most of my memories, I remember what outfit I was wearing at the time. It's sort of distracting, and in a way makes me feel like I'm not fully experiencing the moment because I'm too busy thinking about how I look when I'm experiencing it. It takes up a lot of space in my mind and my memories. Most women I've talked to about this relate to it, while most men haven't understood it at all."

The rise of social media has no doubt contributed to our need to self-objectify. "Because photo-taking is so constant nowadays, many girls and women feel like they have to at all times monitor their appearance and be 'camera ready,'" says Renee Engeln, a professor of psychology at Northwestern University and author of *Beauty Sick*. "We start to see the types of anxieties that used to be limited to celebrities dealing with paparazzi." Plus, in the age of social media, the evaluation and scrutiny that we're trying to manage by monitoring ourselves is no longer just imagined. It's real and quantifiable, in the form of likes, comments, and shares, upping the pressure even more.

"If there's even a slim chance that you have a photo opportunity when you're hanging out with friends or something, it means it's up to you to look as perfect as you possibly can."

Body-image researchers have found that the degree to which we self-objectify is one of the most important predictors of body dissatisfaction, which makes sense: when you base the worth of your body on other people's opinions of it, not only are you much more likely to compare yourself to others in order to gauge your body's attractiveness, but you'll also place a much greater significance on your culture's beauty standards. And that's bad news for everyone, no matter what you look like. Because as Lindsay Kite, body-image researcher and codirector of the nonprofit Beauty Redefined, puts it, "We all fall short of manufactured beauty ideals simply by being humans and not images."

What's sex got to do with it?

Although tabloid gossip columns and various TV makeover shows are doing a fine job on their own coaching women to look at their bodies as objects, there's another factor that's contributing to the objectification of the female body that we need to talk about: the hypersexualization of pop culture. Because not only does the media bombard us with images of gorgeous female bodies, but it also bombards us with images of gorgeous *sexualized* female bodies. "What we used to call soft-core pornography thirty years ago is now mainstream pop culture," Gail Dines, professor emerita of sociology and women's studies at Wheelock College, told me. "Images that you would find in *Playboy* or *Penthouse* are now in Victoria's Secret ads going on buses—they're everywhere."

Plenty of studies have confirmed that the number of sexualized images of women in magazines and ads have skyrocketed. Unfortunately, this increase has little to do with a more open attitude to sex, which becomes obvious when you look at how men are represented in the media compared to women. It's only images of women that have become more sexualized; images of men haven't. And according to a study by sociologists at the State University of New York at Buffalo that compared magazine covers, "In the 2000s, there were ten times more hypersexualized images of women than men, and eleven times more non-sexualized images of men than of women."

Sexualized images of women have become so normalized that we don't question their existence even in contexts that have zero to do with sex. When Instagrammers do their signature butt-popping pose next to local sights on every travel picture, when fashion brands advertise their new gym wear collection by having a model pose seductively with a skipping rope, and when pop stars do the sexy baby face while singing about overcoming obstacles in life, sexy is the new default look.

Sexual objectification vs. sexual empowerment

For many years, the argument that the hypersexualization of pop culture is negatively affecting women and men did not make it into mainstream media or was even actively refused as some kind of antisex fear-mongering in the vein of "We worked too hard to allow women to express their sexuality to now scold them for taking off their clothes." And in contemporary feminism, the difference between sexual objectification and sexual empowerment is still one of the most hotly debated topics, because on a surface level they can look similar. Is that actress's nude spread in a magazine empowering, or is she succumbing to the pressures of a patriarchal society? Is that female pop star's music video pushing boundaries for modern womanhood, or is it just fueling the male gaze? And if our hypersexualized culture is marginalizing women's bodies, does that make every bikini photo, every flirty selfie, every seductive pose on social media *bad*?

Okay, slow down.

Yes, it is a problem that our pop culture as a whole is becoming more sexualized. We should be mad at big brands and corporations for releasing ad campaigns that reduce multifaceted human beings to sex objects. But that does not mean that we should slam individual women (including actresses and pop stars) for posting sexy pics, for two reasons. First, as a principle, it's never cool to blame an individual for acting in line with values that have been given to them by a messed-up system. And second, not every photo or video that is *sexual* is also *sexually objectifying*. The difference lies in agency.

Is the actress reluctantly posing in a men's magazine at the suggestion of her manager, or is she excited about doing the shoot because it's with a photographer whom she admires for their creative vision? Was this sexy bikini selfie posted by a social media account that routinely rates, sexualizes, and scrutinizes women's bodies with no regard to the owners of those bodies, or was it shared by the woman herself?

Sexualized photos themselves are not the problem. A woman's sexuality is one of her many facets that she is allowed to express, however she likes. The problem is that our media landscape shows, values, and celebrates women's sex appeal *more* than any of their other qualities, opinions, or accomplishments.

"I used to think only shallow people worry about the way they look, but now I know it's not a sign of vanity or weakness to have a poor body image—it's a normal, natural response to a brutal culture."

When I grow up . . .

When you grow up as a girl surrounded by sexualized images of women, it changes the way you build your identity. "Adolescence is a time when you begin to question who you are and who you're going to be as an adult," says Gail Dines. "You're wandering around the culture looking for norms about what it means to be female. But since there's only really one dominant image of femininity in this culture, your options are limited: you're either fuckable or invisible. And no adolescent can tolerate being invisible."

In the '50s, the notion of the ideal woman was the perfect housewife who prepares home-cooked dinners for her family of five every night and throws lavish parties in her perfect home to impress her husband's colleagues on the weekend. Sound backwards and deeply sexist? Sure, but today's female ideal is not much better. Today, the ideal women is still above all one thing: hot. She can run a company, she can be a UN humanitarian, she can be an artist, she can be a mom, but the one thing we'll admire her for the most is her looks and her sex appeal. Being desirable is the one nonnegotiable of today's ideal woman. And because of that, women in our culture have no choice but to deeply care about their looks.

The problem with body positivity

Although the digital age has definitely intensified the three major culprits behind our collective body worries—the beauty blast, the objectification of female bodies, and our hypersexualized pop culture—it's not all bad. Social media, in particular, has played a major role in promoting diversity and holding brands, magazines, and film studios accountable for portraying a wider range of bodies and looks. It has also been a huge driver of the body positivity movement, whose goals are to call out narrow beauty ideals and encourage women to love their bodies and see beauty in their "flaws."

Body positivity has done a ton to help shift our culture's media narrative in a better direction, from reducing shame and pointing out the ridiculousness of our society's beauty ideals to increasing awareness that much of what you see in the media is an illusion. But here's the trouble: when it comes to developing a healthy long-term body image, body positivity—in the way that it is commonly understood and presented today—means well but is not giving us the right tools to actually reach that goal. Here's why.

"All bodies are beautiful"

While the main message of "all bodies are beautiful" does address the issue of narrow beauty ideals (the tip of the iceberg), in doing so it also reinforces the core belief that got us into this mess in the first place: that looking (and feeling beautiful) is a prerequisite to happiness. Telling women to "remember that you're beautiful" or that their stretch marks are beautiful is no doubt meant to be consoling and empowering. But it also keeps women's attention fixed on their mirror image—on what they see, how they feel about what they see, and what others think about what they see. It keeps them stuck in the same self-objectifying, appearance-focused thought pattern that's been fueling their insecurities all along. And it keeps them from working toward a long-lasting, healthy relationship with their body, which requires them to step away from the mirror.

"I hate when people tell other people they should be happy with their given bodies and love their flaws. It implies that there is a flaw that needs accepting and leaves no space for people's real and meaningful feelings."

Nude selfies

As we've already discussed, there is nothing wrong with sexualized photos, including nude selfies, but their role as primary symbol for body-image activism is problematic for the same reason as the "all bodies are beautiful" type of slogans. It yet again puts the focus on the female body as an object. As body-image researchers Lindsay and Lexie Kite from Beauty Redefined put it: "The second generation [of body-positive activists] must move beyond the now-stagnant place of body photos with long captions about how those bodies are beautiful and worthy. Of course they are. But women are more than bodies, and we must back that up with the ways we choose to represent and value ourselves and all women, online or otherwise."

CHAPTER 3

OTHER PEOPLE

The media has a huge impact on the way we feel about our bodies, but it's our real-life experiences that really lodge these messages into our subconscious. Whether it's their mom asking with a disapproving look if they really want that second piece of cake, their dad making fun of the neighbor lady's wrinkles, or that time a boy they liked in school called them "horse teeth," many women I interviewed remember the exact moment they started worrying about their weight, their nose, the hair on their arms, or the way their gums show when they smile. Just one or two experiences can so often set the tone for the rest of our life. And just as it's important to become aware of the media's effect on our body image, it's also crucial that we pinpoint these defining moments in our personal lives, to help turn our insecurities from abstract, be-all and end-all clouds that loom over our heads into a clearly defined problem with tangible causes that we can chip away at piece by piece.

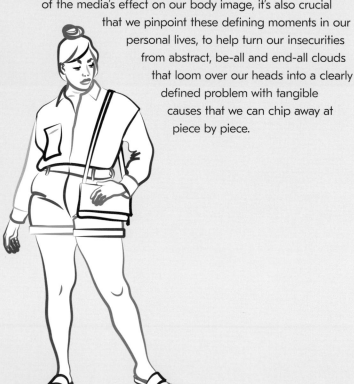

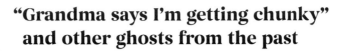

"Grandma says I'm getting chunky" and other ghosts from the past

When I was about five and still blissfully unaware of beauty ideals and societal pressures, I overheard my grandmother telling my mom that I seemed to have gotten "a little chunky." My mom disagreed, but still, I could sense from that interaction that "chunky" was clearly a bad thing, and that I was at least teetering dangerously close to it.

As kids, our personalities, values, and belief systems are like soft, squishy Play-Doh. Every experience, every interaction, and every comment can leave an impression and shape the way we think, feel, and act as grown-ups. If you don't feel great about your body now, chances are you, too, can think of a few not-so-great experiences in your childhood that etched themselves into your memory and set the basis for how you think of your body—like the "chunky" incident did for me. Those experiences don't necessarily have to be outright criticism or even be directed to you at all. Often, it's the little things that stick.

Modeling

As children, we pick up many of beliefs and values from simply observing our parents' and other adults' behavior. Psychologists call this *modeling*. Modeling can affect us in both a positive and a negative way. If your mother constantly criticizes her own body and tells you that she is "not allowed to eat pizza" because she "needs to look good for the summer," you learn that women need to fit a certain standard and that restricting your food helps you do that. If your mother gets complimented on her appearance all the time, you learn that beauty is good and that it leads people to be nice to you. If your dad criticizes women on TV or your brother makes fun of girls at school, you learn that men judge a girl's appearance and that not having the right appearance can lead you to be ridiculed.

On the other hand, if your parents don't criticize their own or other people's bodies and choose food, clothes, and activities based on how much they personally like them rather than how they will affect their weight or looks, you're much more likely to grow up thinking of your looks as a nonissue (although other factors, like the media, may still knock a dent in your confidence).

"My granny was always on diets and talking about food being too 'luscious' and how she shouldn't be eating it. That had an effect on my mom, and I know it definitely made me self-conscious about what I was eating."

Teasing

For a lot of people, being teased about some body part by either a family member or a peer was what made them aware of a "flaw" for the very first time. One woman told me: "I had never even thought about my ears until the boy next door called me 'Smurf ears.' I didn't wear my hair up once all the way until high school."

But is teasing really so bad? "Everyone gets teased about something; it's part of growing up!" said one woman in my survey. Is she right, and are we as a culture getting overly sensitive? Should we tell our past selves and (future) children to just get over it?

> "Throughout my teen years I was told that I was too tall and too thin. I started slouching and walking with my head down because I was so embarrassed, even though it would make my back, shoulders, and neck ache."

My opinion: a big fat no. Just because something is common does not mean it's okay. Both bullying and teasing can have huge negative effects on children, and the line between them can often be blurry. Just because a comment was meant as a joke or even said out of affection does not mean the receiver will understand it that way. So instead of telling girls that it's no big deal, we should encourage them to have compassion—for themselves and for others. Because no, getting teased about some minor aspect of your appearance *shouldn't* be a big deal, but in our looks-obsessed world, it is a big deal.

BULLYING FACTS

- Around one-third of girls report having been bullied online or at school.

- Most bullying occurs in middle school, a highly defining time for children's social and emotional development.

- By far the most common thing both girls and boys are bullied about is their weight or other aspects of their appearance.

- Bullying during childhood has been linked to increased rates of depression, anxiety, and eating disorders in adulthood and, no surprise here, low self-esteem.

"At school I got called an 'albino' because of my very pale skin and hair. I was so embarrassed about it and didn't know what else to do, so I just tried to ignore it. But for a while it's what I thought everyone thought when they saw me."

"I hate it when people say, 'You're short,' like it's some kind of deficiency, or as if maybe I hadn't noticed. I try not to get irritated. My height is not a choice, but being a jerk is."

Intentional criticism from adults

My parents never commented on my looks in a negative way, but I did have two very outspoken grandmothers who clearly believed it was their duty to inform me of any pre-adolescent weight gain, perhaps in case I hadn't noticed. I remember very clearly when I was thirteen, one of them sat me down to say, "You used to be so slim, what happened?" (puberty) and to recommend I eat fewer sweets. Plenty of women in my survey had a similar story to share of a relative outright body-shaming them as a kid.

If you ask those adults about their intention, they would no doubt tell you that they were doing it out of love and concern. They know it's a superficial world out there and being attractive is what counts. So in an intervention-style tough-love effort, they are trying to make sure you are aware of the problem and motivate you to change, just like they might urge you to study more if your grades are lacking. But here's the thing: not fitting the beauty ideal is not even slightly comparable to not acing seventh-grade math.

> "When I had severe adolescent acne, my parents were more upset about it than I was, dragging me to various dermatologists and once grounding me when they discovered I wasn't using my Retin-A cream. At one point during a confrontation about it, my mother cried and said she worried I'd never be successful or loved if I didn't get my face 'under control.'"

We may not feel great about a bad grade, but in our culture there is nothing inherently shameful about it. As a thirteen-year-old, I would have had no problem telling my friend—while rolling my eyes—"My mom is making me study, ugh." But I would have never been able to say, "My mom told me I should eat less because I am getting fat," because there is so much shame attached to being or looking different. Even twelve-year-olds are fully aware that the way you look is a crucial, if not the most important, value for women in our society.

By "confronting" young girls about some aspect of their appearance, we are not simply giving them harmless tips, we are directly tearing into their already-fragile feelings of self-worth and adding yet another layer of shame.

Besides, making children feel bad about their weight in an effort to motivate them to lose weight can seriously backfire. Studies have shown that, if anything, weight-based criticism leads to binge eating and weight *gain*. For example, one recent study found that girls who are told that they are "too fat" at age ten are 66 percent more likely to be obese by age nineteen (and that's after controlling for their initial weight).

"At twelve I got glasses. My mother could be very harsh (which was how she was raised), and I clearly remember the hurt and shame I felt when she said that I should only use my glasses to read but take them off at all other times, because no one liked a girl with glasses."

REFLECTION QUESTIONS

When was the earliest time you remember being concerned with your appearance?

Did you attempt to improve your appearance as a child? How about as a teenager?

Did your parents ever outwardly criticize your weight?

Did your parents ever outwardly criticize another aspect of your appearance?

Was there someone in your family who always got a lot of compliments on their looks? How did that make you feel?

Did you witness your mother (or other close female family members) being concerned or preoccupied with her appearance?

Were you ever aware of your family trying to modify what or how much you ate or exercised?

Did you get bullied by other kids because of your appearance?

Were there any comments that your friends made about your appearance that stuck with you?

Have you ever been body-shamed?

"I was sitting in my car at a stoplight the other day, and the guy in front of me had a sticker on his back window that said, 'No fat chicks.' I think it's hard not to feel shame as a woman in our society when stuff like that is everywhere. I tell myself that that guy is probably just a jerk, but it only helps so much."

"I had friends in high school who said a nose job would take me from a 6 out of 10 to an 8 out of 10. A coworker told me that in his culture, my nose would be called a beak. I have friends who say things like, 'So what, you have other beautiful features,' implying that though it may be ugly, I can put my focus elsewhere. These comments stay with me, and I have to actively fight against those echoing voices in my head."

"Once when my belly was bloated someone asked me whether I really wanted to have that drink. I just said, 'Yes I want that drink,' but it did hurt that people apparently thought I was pregnant just because I am not skinny or X-shaped."

"My first boyfriend ridiculed my small breasts, saying our babies would have snack-size feeds. I dumped him and went on to successfully breastfeed both my babies until they were two years old, which was very healing for me."

"I haven't been body-shamed, partly because I've lived a sheltered life, but also because for most of it, I've been so worried about being criticized for my looks that I avoid any possible situation where it might arise—and missing out on all kinds of opportunities in the process."

BEYOND
BEAUTIFUL
TOOLBOX

A typology of body-shamers (and how to clap back)

Of course, it's not just interpersonal experiences in our childhood that affect our body image—for most people, adulthood too is rife with moments that test our body image, courtesy of callous exes, catty friends, and random strangers.

Here's a typology of the most common body-shamers and how to handle them.

The concern-trolling relative

Parents, grandparents, aunts, and uncles who are trying to make sure you're maximizing your chances in life by conforming to beauty standards.

Says things like:

"You should stop working out so much; you don't want to start looking all manly."

"This veganism thing isn't working out for you; you're losing your curves."

"Maybe you should try a spinning class. I heard it's great for weight loss."

Clapback:

Respond in a clear, firm tone: "Thank you for your input, but I am happy with my body as is."

The "just kidding" friend

Members of your closest friend group who've gotten in the habit of trashing each other as a form of endearment.

Says things like:

"Look at you and your itty-bitty boobs."

"Move your fat ass over here."

"We can't all have toothpick legs like you."

Clapback:

Say, "Look, I know you are not trying to be mean, but I'm trying to steer clear from body-related negativity these days."

The "fair game"

Acquaintances, colleagues, and people you just met who believe that it's fair game to make fun of features that are considered desirable according to society's beauty ideal.

Says things like:

"Oh my god, your boobs are enormous."

"You have like zero body fat; eat something!"

"What's the air like up there?"

Clapback:

Ask, "Sorry, can you repeat that?" with a completely straight face. Forcing people to repeat an offensive comment tends to make them reconsider; in either case, the "joke" will lose its momentum and fall flat.

The ignorant professional

Sales assistants, hairstylists, personal trainers, and other people at work giving you "helpful" advice that you didn't ask for.

Says things like:

"Pleats have a super slimming effect on fuller figures."

"Have you ever considered sclerotherapy for your spider veins? We can do that in-house."

"Barbell squats will help add some curves to your frame."

Clapback:

Respond with matching factuality: "I'm not interested in slimming my figure/getting rid of my spider veins/adding curves to my frame, thank you."

The troll

Shames your appearance on social media photos, can be anything from pseudofriendly to blatantly offensive.

Says things like:

"I am not trying to be mean, but that outfit really doesn't work for your body."

"Girl, you need a better bra!"

"Wow! I hadn't noticed you gained weight."

Clapback:

Ignore, delete, block if necessary.

The callous lover

Whether out of ignorance, a misguided attempt at humor, or to subtly shame us into conforming to their preferences, body-shaming hurts twice as much when it comes from a person who's seen us naked.

Says things like:

"You almost have broader shoulders than me!"

"Your little chubby rolls are so cute."

"You could be a lingerie model if your boobs were bigger."

Clapback:

Silence, then: "Okay, I'm going to let this one slide. But for future reference, I'm really not a fan of body-shaming."

How has your upbringing influenced the way you feel about your body today?

"My mom is OBSESSED with weight, and I am pretty sure that her obsession is the source of the majority of my weight hang-ups. We have this joke in my family that my mom says goodbye by saying, 'See you later. Remember you're fat.'"

"My parents did not raise me to think I didn't look good, but that didn't stop me from having that idea."

"My family would regularly comment on how my nose looks so much like my father's (which is big and flat) and how I had inherited my auntie's wide hips and flat chest. They felt insecure about these family traits and decided so should I."

"I was born with crooked fingers but I have honestly never been bothered by them because my parents never made any sort of deal about them. My cousin also has crooked fingers and he feels very self-conscious about them, and I am sure it's because his mother always made comments about how he should move his hand out of pictures and how he doesn't need to worry when it comes to finding a girlfriend because girls couldn't care less about a guy's fingers—stuff like that. I feel so bad for him."

"My mom had an eating disorder and, weirdly, it encouraged me to develop a better relationship with my body and food, to not be like her."

"I have three sisters, and we were raised to compete with each other. To this day, each of us has massive insecurities born from my parents telling us the other was better looking, smarter, or more popular."

"My upbringing has definitely had a positive influence on how I feel about my body now. My parents always emphasized the importance of health, good food, and being independent and would encourage my brother and me to play sports, go camping, or just roam around outside. My family has a history of eating disorders, so my mother didn't want me to go down the same path."

"I am honestly so grateful that my aunt (who raised me) put zero focus on the way anyone looked. In comparison to my friends, I feel so much less insecure about my flaws and it's not because I have fewer; they just don't seem particularly consequential. My aunt once gained a lot of weight quickly due to medication and all she said was 'Time to go shopping!' And when she came off the medication and lost the weight a year later, there was no celebrating or 'Thank god I look like myself again' or anything."

"Whenever we were watching a movie, my dad would always pick apart how the actresses looked. From a young age that made me believe that a woman's value is in how she looks—that if she's ugly, she's not as valuable as the pretty ones. Rationally, I can say to myself, 'That's not true!' But there's always still this voice in my head saying, 'Do whatever you can to look perfect.'"

"I was raised LDS (Mormon) and had it constantly drilled into my head that 'Modest is hottest.' In Mormon culture, what you wear often gets tied to your worth. I no longer practice, but I sometimes still feel the shame that I felt as a twelve-year-old girl being told that my shorts were too short, and that they would make boys think inappropriate thoughts. How absurd is that? I am not responsible for, nor am I capable of controlling, the thoughts and opinions of those around me."

Why we need to change how we talk about our bodies

Besides body-shaming, the number one way that our inter-personal relationships reinforce a negative body image is through body talk. You know the type: "Ugh, my butt looks enormous in these jeans. I need to start working out again." "At least your butt is nice and round, mine looks like a pancake." "What are you talking about, your butt is fine. I wish I had your body-fat percentage." "Well, I can take some of your fat if you trade me some boobs."

Conversations like these, consisting of back-and-forth complaining about our own appearance, mutual reassurance, and discussion of potential fixes, have become a staple communication ritual in our culture. Studies have shown that body talk happens across the board, regardless of age or body size. One Australian study that had women aged eighteen to forty report body talk as it happened in real time found that more than a quarter of all of their social interactions during the one week the experiment ran contained some form of body talk. "[Fat talk] is not just accepted but expected—it's the social norm for women to talk in this way about their bodies. Other studies have shown that it's basically weird if you don't engage in fat talk," says Dr. Jacqueline Mills, the lead researcher of that study, in an article for *Psychlopaedia*.

Body talk is so common because in the moment it makes you feel better, especially when that other person admits to being insecure about their appearance as well. Body talk is also a way of being intimate with someone else, which helps us bond. Plus, in a culture that places so much importance on our female appearance, it's only logical that women *think* about their appearance frequently and thus it is also a common topic in their conversations.

But according to Renee Engeln, the prevalence of body talk is not just a simple reflection of our collective body dissatisfaction; it also further promotes it. "When we disparage our bodies in conversations with other women, we do three things. First, we implicitly give other people permission to talk about our bodies (or other women's bodies) in that same disrespectful way. Second, we direct other women's attention to their own appearance. Finally, we feed into the notion that body-hatred is a normal part of being a woman, that it's something to bond over instead of something to actively work against."

"I have amazingly supportive girlfriends: we go swimming naked together, change in front of each other, share our journeys, and their words are slowly replacing all the negative comments, body-shaming, and teasing I experienced in high school."

REFLECTION QUESTIONS

How prevalent is body talk within your different peer groups (your close and casual friends, colleagues, family members, and so on)?

What social function do you think talking about your body serves in each case?

Does body talk make you feel better or worse about the way you look?

Are there any comments that people have made about your appearance that have stuck with you?

In your friend group, do you tease each other about your appearance?

Five essential rules for (self-) talking about your body

So, should we not talk about our insecurities at all? Should we just grin and bear it? No, of course not! If you are lucky enough to have friends that you trust, being open and honest about your struggle is a great thing because it reduces the shame that underlies all body worries, not just for you, but also for everyone else that is a part of the conversation. To make sure your sharing session isn't inadvertently fueling body-hate (your friends' or your own), stick to a few ground rules (and try to also keep these in mind when it comes to your internal self-talk):

Rule 1

Focus on the internal rather than the external aspects of your insecurities. Rather than dwelling on all the physical details of your self-perceived flaws, focus on how they make you feel, how they affect your life, and where these insecurities may come from.

INSTEAD OF "I hate the way my hips dip out, then in, then out again. I wish that bit of fat from my belly pooch could just go move to that dip in my hips."

SAY "I feel insecure about the way my hips look, because in the media all you see is celebrity bodies with perfectly smooth silhouettes in tight bodycon dresses."

Rule 2

When your friend tells you about her insecurities, don't try to match or one-up her. It may be the protocol that you've internalized for these types of conversations, but try your hardest to resist the urge. Listen to her story and offer consolation, but don't compare her insecurities with your own.

INSTEAD OF "That little bit of extra skin is nothing— look at my batwings!"

SAY "Your arms look totally fine to me but as a woman living in the same looks-obsessed world as you do, I understand these types of feelings."

Rule 3

Don't present your body insecurities as facts— they are feelings.

INSTEAD OF "I am hideous."

SAY "I feel hideous."

Rule 4

Train yourself to use an objective perspective when talking about your insecurities.

INSTEAD OF "I look like a twelve-year-old boy."

SAY "I am flat-chested."

Rule 5

Don't say you *need* or *can't* do something because of the way your body looks (unless you are literally seven feet tall and want to be an Air Force fighter pilot).

INSTEAD OF "I can't wear short dresses because I have the ugliest knees."

SAY "I feel very self-conscious about my knees so I keep them covered up."

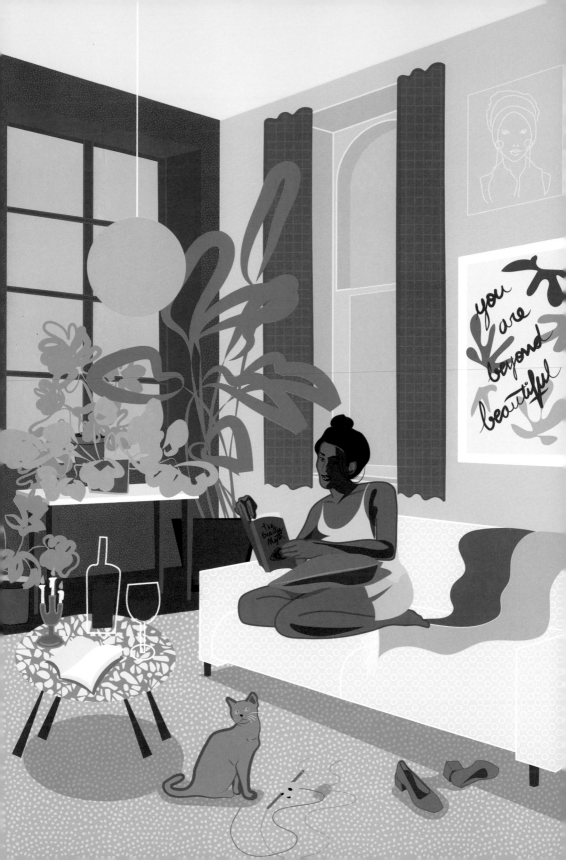

PART II

REWRITE YOUR MENTAL SCRIPT

CHAPTER 4

SELF-PERCEPTION

One of the very first things that stood out to me when I started interviewing women for this book is that a less-than-ideal body image often goes hand in hand with an intense level of body awareness. No matter whom I asked, from my eight-year-old neighbor to my eighty-year-old grandma, every single woman could tell me *exactly* what was wrong with her body and describe her "flaws" to an impressive level of detail. "My hips are too wide for my body." "My torso has an odd shape." "My left nostril does this weird thing when I smile." "My jaw muscles stick out too much, which throws my whole face off balance." Et cetera, et cetera.

After years of scrutinizing our mirror image, it seems like we've all come up with a clear story line about our bodies—a story that we keep telling ourselves over and over and that we carry around as if it's based on stone-cold facts, when really, it's "inspired by true events" at best. The goal of this chapter is to show you why your evaluations of your body might not be quite as black-and-white as you think, so you can start firing unhelpful beliefs from their cushy long-term spot in your brain and ultimately replace them with some fresh and body-positive new ones.

Exactly how pretty am I?

When I was in sixth grade, my whole grade collectively decided that we should all work together to create a top three "most beautiful list" for every single body part: most beautiful lips, most beautiful hair, most beautiful legs, and so on. Looking back, I feel equal parts amused and horrified by how seriously we all took this. I also wonder what our motivation was. Part of it must have been a form of social power play and/or fishing for compliments, but I think there was more to it. For several days we spent our breaks walking around, examining each other from head to toe, and writing down our "observations." We made sure to present our faces with a neutral expression and reminded each other not to award our friends extra points. We wanted to be objective, because we wanted accurate results.

I remembered this story when I stumbled upon an essay by writer Haley Nahman about how even as a kid she was so obsessed with pinpointing her "true" appearance, she'd use every reflective surface to check herself out. "I wasn't vain; I was curious," she writes. And really, how could she not be curious? In a world that teaches girls and women that a) their looks are their most defining quality and b) that anyone's looks can be easily quantified into a single number, how could any one of us not have an intense need to know exactly what *our* number is?

In the era of "Hot or Not," photo or no photo, and swipe right or swipe left, we're all totally used to the idea that when it comes to attractiveness, we all exist somewhere on a spectrum and, bar any major physical changes, we're stuck at our level. However, one of the biggest revelations I had while writing this book is that people with a healthy body image tend to have a much more fluid perception of their appearance. One woman whom I'd asked whether she ever thought she looked bad in a photo said, "Definitely! Just last week my husband took a photo of me and I looked awful." I then asked, "So how do bad photos like that make you feel?" "Oh, that wasn't a bad photo, I really looked bad that day. But sometimes I also look great!"

"Self-perception is a zoo."

Jen Sincero

Ultimately, the goal of a healthy body image is, of course, to understand that it doesn't matter whether you are a 6 out of 10 or an 8 out of 10 according to society's beauty ideals. But I think a baby step toward that can be to recognize that your attractiveness is not fixed, but variable. We can all look better or worse, depending on a huge number of factors. Our level of attractiveness is not an inherent quality of ourselves. One bad photo is not proof that we are ugly, and one good photo does not mean we are hot shit. Or as Haley Nahman put it: "Maybe there is no definitive answer as to whether I'm pretty, adorable, or grotesque. Maybe I'm all of those things and more."

"Whenever I see a photo of myself, I try to 'objectively' rate my attractiveness on a scale, and that rating often determines how I feel about myself for the rest of the day. The ratings fluctuate a lot, of course, because so much of it depends on things like the lighting and the angle."

What you see in the mirror is not real

If you were online in 2013, you probably saw the Dove Real Beauty Sketches campaign in which FBI forensic artist Gil Zamora drew sketches of women's faces, based on how they described themselves. He then drew a second sketch based on how one of the other participants saw her. At the end we saw the two sketches side by side and, in every single case, the difference was huge. In the drawing that was based on the woman's self-description, she looked tired and unhappy, certain features were exaggerated, wrinkles were more pronounced. The second sketch was always the more attractive one.

Now, it's easy to chalk up these results to plain politeness. Of course, people weren't going to trash someone else's appearance with a camera in front of their face. And perhaps the artist was at least subconsciously trying to make the second sketches nicer looking than the first one. But then you saw the women standing in front of the two sketches, and it turns out, politeness had nothing to do with it. The second sketch—the one that was based on a stranger's viewpoint—always bore a much greater resemblance to the women's actual faces.

The message of the study is one that psychologists have known for years: women judge their own attractiveness not just more negatively than other people do, but also less *accurately*.

Why you are probably overestimating the size of your body

You may have heard that people with eating disorders often have a distorted view of their bodies and see themselves as bigger than they really are. But did you know that there is plenty of evidence that shows that even women who have never been diagnosed with an eating disorder have a tendency to overestimate their size? Yep, surprised me, too.

In one classic study, participants had to adjust light beams to match the estimated width of their cheeks, thighs, waist, and hips. The results: women overestimated the width of all four body parts by an average of 25 percent. That is a lot!

In another study, women were asked to digitally adjust a distorted full-frontal image of their body to match their real body as closely as possible. Again, women overestimated the size of their bodies across the board. Another key finding of that same study was that the women's BMI was not in the slightest related to how much they overestimated their size or whether they did at all. Women of all shapes and sizes see their bodies as bigger than they really are.

Perhaps the clearest evidence that something's off with the way we perceive our own bodies comes from a recent study where women had to rate the attractiveness of different computer-generated bodies. The clue was that some of the bodies were shown with the participant's own face. And, you guessed it: all women consistently rated bodies with a stranger's face as more attractive than bodies with their own face. Talk about a double standard!

But why does this happen? We spend an average of fifty minutes per day staring at our reflection. Shouldn't we know what we look like? What's happening in our brain that makes us perceive our own bodies so much more negatively (and less clearly) than other people's bodies?

Un-skew your perception:
The "one thing" habit

One of the most effective things you can do to up how you feel about the way you look takes less than three seconds: find one thing that you like about your appearance every single time you look at yourself in a mirror from now on.

Old habits die hard, so don't worry if your eyes jump straight to your "flaws." Let them. But after that, direct your gaze to something you're happy with, whether it's your on-point eye makeup or the way your boobs look in that dress. Acknowledge it, then move on.

To figure that out, a group of researchers came up with an eye-tracking experiment, where women who had been diagnosed with an eating disorder as well as healthy control subjects were shown various pictures of their own and other people's bodies, while their eye gaze was monitored. Participants who suffered from an eating disorder looked at their own bodies in a very particular way: they kept their eyes fixed on body parts they considered unattractive and pretty much ignored the rest of their body. They did the exact opposite when it came to the other people's bodies: they kept their gaze on what they would later label the attractive parts and glossed over the rest.

Now, although this study was conducted with participants suffering from an eating disorder, psychologists believe that the same attentional bias is what's behind all those studies that have demonstrated how even healthy women misperceive the way their body looks to a hefty degree. Think about it: when you walk past a mirror, where do your eyes go? Do you focus on the bits you know you like or do you stare at your flaws? I know for me, especially when I'm not feeling great, I zoom in straight to my thighs or my arms, nothing else. When I see a picture of myself, I immediately check if my legs seem fat or my arms chubby—the rest I barely notice.

Researchers believe that the reason we do this is actually pretty simple: in cognitive psychology it is well known that humans are programmed to pay attention to things they have strong feelings about or consider a threat. And in a culture that equates beauty with value and lovability, "flaws" pose a threat. The problem is, of course, if you only ever pay attention to what you consider your least attractive or biggest body parts while ignoring the rest, your perception of these parts takes over the picture you have of your entire body, and you'll think you're less attractive overall or bigger than you really are.

Why you hate the way you look in photos

We've all been there: scrolling mindlessly through your social media feeds when you get a notification that someone tagged you in a photo—and it's a *bad* one. Whatever mood you were in before is now replaced by a gut-wrenching mix of anxiety, shame, and sadness. "That's what I look like? And all this time I've been walking around thinking I am somewhat decent-looking. Turns out that's all been a lie; I am actually hideous."

"I absolutely hate it when people take pictures of me. I do not recognize myself in pictures. That's not me, that's not how I feel I look, and that's not how I look in the mirror. I know I am pretty, and then suddenly come these photos, challenging my perception of myself. No, thank you!"

Most of us are well aware of the enormous impact just one bad photo can have on our mood and go to great lengths to protect ourselves from the looming emotional pain. "The fuss most of my friends make when someone wants to take a photo is absurd," said one woman in my survey. "There will be people who refuse to be in it, have to stand in the back or in the middle to hide their arms or whatever, or make everyone wait because they need to get changed. It's like, 'You were fine all day with everyone seeing what you look like and now you are freaking out?'"

But there is actually a perfectly simply explanation why the majority of people dislike themselves in photos, even when they have no problem with what they see in the mirror. It is the same reason why we hate hearing our own voice. Both our recorded voice and our image in a photo seem strange and unpleasant to us because they're simply not what we are used to. Our voice sounds different on a recording than it does when we hear our own voice when we speak because the sound waves travel through a different pathway. Our face and body look different in photos than they do in the mirror because most people subconsciously pose in a certain flattering way in front of the mirror and because your mirror image is inverted from left to right.

When the way we look in a photo doesn't match the mental image we have of ourselves, the differences become exaggerated and our face seems distorted and just plain strange. Plenty of studies have shown that people much prefer photos of themselves when they are flipped horizontally and therefore look closer to what they are used to seeing in the mirror.

It's all about familiarity. That is also why people whose job involves being on camera (public figures, reporters, actors, and so on) tend to be much more comfortable seeing photos or videos of themselves. It's not that they necessarily find themselves that much more attractive than the rest of us—their mental image of themselves has simply aligned to what they've seen over and over again on camera.

How do you feel about the way you look in photos?

"I've come to accept that photos aren't a true representation of what I look like. In the words of Ani DiFranco: 'I don't take good pictures, cuz I have the kind of beauty that moves.'"

"I remember getting into trouble at school for refusing to have a school photo taken. I was told I was being selfish and difficult but actually I couldn't bear to see an image of myself."

"I am eighty years old and have the advantage of being able to look back over a lifetime of photos. Photos where I thought I looked awful look pretty good to me today."

"One side of my nose is bigger than the other and my smile is crooked, so I try as hard as possible to face the camera from my left side."

"I detest the way I look in photographs and avoid them or deliberately sabotage my appearance (pulling faces or ducking out of the shot at the last minute). I have no comprehension of the selfie: why, why, would you want pictures of yourself out there where people would see and judge them?"

"When I post a selfie, it's one of at least a dozen or so that I took in order to get the right angle, lighting, and pose, and my facial structure and size have been edited. I have been called out for making the same exact facial expression in every photo—but it's just the only one I think looks good."

"I don't do selfies. I am startled enough by how I look in store windows."

BEYOND
BEAUTIFUL
TOOLBOX

Bad photo emergency: How to deal in five steps

Consider these five steps your first response plan of action for the next bad photo emergency. Your goal here is not to convince yourself that you actually look great, but to turn down the intensity of your feelings and recognize the photo for what it is: a bad representation of yourself that is of no consequence.

Step 1: Acknowledge that you are likely seeing yourself in an overly critical way

The unfamiliarity effect we discussed on page 75 is just one of the many reasons why you shouldn't pay too much attention to your own judgment of a photo. Remember how the various studies on this showed that women a) consistently overestimate their body size and b) have a tendency to focus only on their worst parts, which then taints their judgment of their whole appearance? When you feel a strong negative reaction to a photo, it is very likely that you are not looking at yourself in a balanced way.

Step 2: Remember that everyone can look better and worse

Physical beauty is not a fixed value, and one bad photo does not prove that you are unattractive. We are all capable of looking amazing and awful, both in photos and in real life, depending on a huge number of factors like lighting, angles, makeup, the time of day, and so on. Even super-models take bad photos.

Step 3: Get angry

Remind yourself of the reason for your strong reaction. You believe that looking bad is a big deal because that's what you've been taught all of your life by big corporations and misguided value systems—and that's messed up.

Step 4: Have compassion

According to Lexie and Lindsay Kite, one of the most important things to do in a situation that seriously disrupts your body image is to be kind to yourself. Have compassion for yourself, just like you would have compassion for every other woman who has been made to feel terrible about herself because of stupid societal ideals. Allow yourself to experience these feelings, but also understand that they will pass.

Step 5: Redirect your attention to the positive memory this photo captures

End on a high note by taking a moment to focus on a positive aspect that this photo represents. What were you doing when this photo was taken? What were you feeling? Were you having fun with friends? Were you exploring a cool place? Were you about to eat a delicious plate of pasta? A photo can just represent a moment in time instead of being an inquisition into your attractiveness in that moment.

CHAPTER 5

BEAUTY STANDARDS

From "curves in all the right places" to flawless, ageless, hairless skin: In this chapter we'll take an in-depth look at exactly where our current beauty ideals come from, because knowledge is power. We need to understand that the standards we're wasting so much energy over are not objective, higher laws that accurately summarize our fellow human beings' preferences, but often simply leftovers of age-old beliefs, artificially created as clever marketing ploys from businesses, or are otherwise arbitrary and plain absurd.

Feel free to roll your eyes, get offended, and get angry—all of these are helpful emotions. Because once you're angry, you've already crossed the biggest hurdle: you know exactly how nonsensical and wrong our society's messages about beauty are. According to body-image expert Thomas F. Cash, the next step is getting to a point where you are so over them, you just tune them out—where seeing another sexist, discriminatory image or hearing an offensive comment still makes you angry but no longer affects your self-esteem. You probably have this exact attitude when it comes to other popular opinions that you don't share, like when you overhear someone ranting about man-hating feminists. You know exactly how wrong they are, so their remarks just roll right off your back.

Hot bodies through history

Although most women I know (myself included) have their fair share of above-the-neck insecurities, our bodies are clearly our Achilles' heels. Partially that may be due to the fact that in our culture, a woman's physical attractiveness is tied to her sexual appeal, which makes our bodies subject to closer scrutiny than our faces. But another important factor is also that until very recently, the level of diversity we would see in the media in terms of body shapes and sizes was essentially zero.

In 1990, author and activist Naomi Wolf coined the term "the official body" to highlight how—with very few exceptions—the bodies of women in the public eye, from politicians to daytime talk show hosts, were so similar, they could easily share the same wardrobe.

Now, almost thirty years later, feminist and diversity issues have reached the mainstream discourse, yet the portrayal of women's bodies in the media has barely changed. Except for a few plus-size supermodels and pop stars, the vast majority of women in the public eye still have that standard size-2 or size-4 body. Young girls *still* grow up in a world where most of their female idols and role models, including actresses, TV personalities, and entrepreneurs— those who represent success and beauty—have the official body. So how could they not consider it the gold standard?

Western female body ideals

The first step to pushing the official body off its high horse is understanding that what we consider attractive today is only the latest iteration of a long line of body ideals throughout history. Since the '90s, Western body ideals have stayed relatively stable (except for a few add-ons, which we'll talk about later), but before that, just in thepast century, what people thought of as the perfect body varied considerably from one decade to the next.

PRE-20TH CENTURY

We know from literature and art that from at least the seventeenth until the twentieth century, the ideal female body was Rubenesque: voluptuous, with a rounded belly and full breasts and hips, like the naked ladies you see in Baroque paintings.

EARLY 20TH CENTURY

In the 1890s, the illustrator Dana Charles Gibson created the Gibson girl, which became the archetype of the modern American woman. The Gibson girl was buxom and hippy like her Rubenesque predecessor, but considered more fragile, with a thin, long neck and an intense hourglass figure, thanks to a corset.

1920s

In the Roaring Twenties (at the tail end of the first wave of feminism), young women wanted to break with conventional norms. They swapped their corsets and full-length skirts for loose, short dresses and bound their chests to achieve the skinny, curveless body shape that was all the rage at the time—the complete opposite of the exaggerated ultracurvy ideal of previous decades.

1940s AND 1950s

After World War II, traditional values were on the rise again, and the glamorous housewife with an hourglass figure became the new female ideal. Many women wore girdles and corsets on a daily basis and sales of weight gainers (pills or tonics promising to help you "add attractive pounds and inches") were booming.

1960s AND 1970s

In the 1960s, young people started to rebel against their conservative parents, the second wave of feminism started, and the explosion of youth culture brought us hippies, mods, and it-girls. The thin, androgynous body ideal of the time was a reflection of this new cultural standard of youth and rebellion, and it remained stable all the way through the 1970s.

1980s

The 1980s was the decade of Jane Fonda, Jazzercise, and a new female ideal: the powerful career woman. The ideal body was still slim, but no longer as emaciated as in the 1960s and 1970s, because unlike ever before, women now wanted their bodies to reflect strength.

1990s

Thanks to Kate Moss and the grunge aesthetic, the 1990s gave rise to the "waif" look, the ideal of the extremely thin, pale, and young-looking woman. The average weight of models dropped considerably to a place where it has stayed ever since. At the same time, big boobs became popular, no doubt thanks to *Baywatch*, and the rate of breast augmentations in the US went through the roof.

NOW

These days, we still value a low body-fat percentage, but on top of that we now also need two more things to qualify as body-beautiful: a large butt and muscle definition.

But things are improving, right?

Many people believe that compared to previous decades, our body ideals nowadays are less discriminatory and more attainable, and that our media landscape is more inclusive and more diverse, too. Wishful thinking or reality?

BUT . . . PLUS-SIZE MODELS!

Yes, we now have plus-size top models who grace high-fashion magazines and runways, but in the grand scheme of things, they are still very much the exception.

More importantly, just because plus-size models can weigh more does not mean that their shape is any more attainable than that of straight-sized models. A photographer told me that body contouring (using liposuction, fat transfer procedures, or implants) is common among plus-size models because few women naturally possess the specific fat distribution that is required. On top of that, at photo shoots, fat suits, padding, and shapewear will often be used to create that perfectly balanced and smooth silhouette.

Including one token plus-size model with perfect proportions in a shoot with a bunch of straight-sized models is better than no diversity at all, but only barely. If we want real diversity, we need to aim higher: for a full and equal representation of all sizes *and* body types.

"'Diversity' is such a catchphrase these days but, as far as I can see, diversity does not seem to have a place when we speak about the female body. Models with different body shapes, plus-size models, mature models, etc. are still only used in a token gesture of diversity on runways or in magazines, but society's standards don't seem to budge."

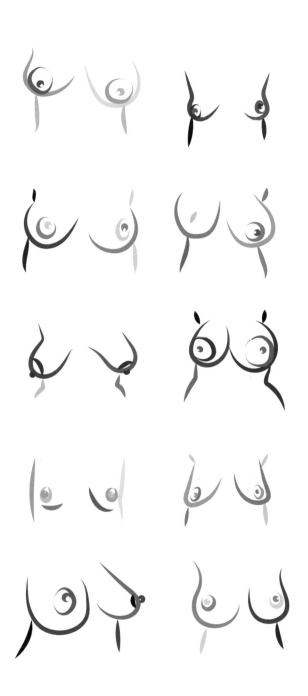

BUT . . . STRONG IS THE NEW SKINNY!

Many people also think of the big butt and "strong is the new skinny" trends as positive developments that have loosened our culture's obsession with "thinner is better" and made our body ideal more attainable to the average woman. However, as much as that is a nice thought, it's a fallacy.

The fact that big butts have become a mainstream trend, unfortunately, doesn't come with a greater appreciation for an allover higher fat percentage. We may be into big butts now, but we still want a tiny waist, thighs that don't touch, and no cellulite, please!

And even though after all these years of women's exercise being about aerobics and one-pound weights, it may seem like a huge win that women now want to get strong. But that new goal has also given rise to a whole new set of insecurities that weren't a thing just a decade ago. You're thin? Okay, but you better not be skinny-fat. Your stomach is flat? Great, but do you have any definition in your abs? You have slim legs? Okay, but what about your glutes?

If "strong" and "curvy" were real alternatives to our existing skinny ideal, that *would* be good news. But as it stands, they are simply add-on criteria that have pushed the female body ideal even further out of reach.

A STRAW OF HOPE

If the fact that—despite all of the public rhetoric about diversity—our body ideals have only proceeded to become *more* rigid in the past decade depresses you, consider this: if you compare how our society's body preferences have shifted in the past, you'll see that new ideals are usually the polar opposite of whatever came before. Now, I don't want to jinx anything, but it's not unthinkable that by the '20s (the 2020s) we'll finally have had enough of all of this rigidity and seeing nothing but lean, sculpted bodies "with curves in all the right places," and our body ideal will be no ideal at all—just pure individuality. Wouldn't that be nice?

What about male body ideals?

Although poor body image is by no means an exclusively female issue, it is safe to say that, overall, the male body-image experience is in a less dire place. Although male and female obesity rates are at a similar level in the US, men report much less dissatisfaction with their bodies, no matter their weight, and are less likely to start a diet than women are. Less than 10 percent of eating disorder sufferers are male, and only around 9 percent of cosmetic surgery procedures are done on men. However, the stats are starting to look bleaker for men, too, and when we examine how the ideal male body has evolved over the past century, that's really no surprise.

Up until the twentieth century, being overweight was a status symbol, because it signaled you had the cash to keep yourself well fed. But once the 1930s rolled around, and the average person had access to Hollywood movies, men everywhere started to prefer a slightly trimmer look, which remained the ideal all the way up until the 1980s. Think Sean Connery's Bond. By today's standards, this slim but not ripped look, with plenty of chest hair, would barely make it as a before pic in fitness magazines.

The skinny, androgynous rocker emerged as an alternative ideal in the 1960s, but average-sized Bond and other Hollywood stars were still on screen, which kept the skinny ideal from going mainstream. Then in 1978, Christopher Reeve became the new Superman and the first one to pack a ton of muscle. By the time the 1980s hit, the bodybuilding craze was in full force. Guys were pumping iron and loading up on protein to look like Arnold Schwarzenegger or Rocky, and steroids became a real problem.

In the 1990s and early 2000s, the craze flattened a bit, and the ideal body swerved from as-big-as-possible to still muscly, but ultralean (think Brad Pitt in *Fight Club*). That body ideal has stayed pretty much consistent, with the addition of a new fitness surge, this time powered by social media. Gym memberships are rising again—and with it male-body dissatisfaction.

You look fine down there, really!

A great thing about the increasing public discourse about body image is that women everywhere are becoming more comfortable talking about their insecurities. But while more of us now may be fine discussing our cellulite or acne, one body part has stayed off-limits: our vulvas.

In the survey that I ran for this book, many women admitted feeling embarrassed about the way they look "down there," about feeling inhibited during sex, and even skipping gynecologist appointments. One woman wrote: "This is so private and I could never actually talk to anyone about it, but I feel very self-conscious about my labia minora, and I am considering plastic surgery just to make me look normal down there." In 2016, labiaplasty was the fastest growing type of surgery in the US, and psychologists believe that it's no coincidence this is happening as porn is becoming more available.

"We should all hang around more with other naked people. There are more 'normals' than you've ever imagined."

Not only has porn put vulvas on the same list as butts, breasts, and every other body part that has a right and a wrong way of looking, but it has also seriously skewed our perception of what's normal by only showing a specific type of vulva. And that lack of vulva diversity, researchers at the University of Amsterdam believe, is a big problem: "Labia minora vary greatly in size, shape, and color. However, in most media that depict women's vulvas (erotic magazines, women's magazines, internet, porn movies), labia minora are not protruding the labia majora. These images are either digitally manipulated or show models that have undergone a labia minora reduction or women who naturally have smaller labial size, and therefore do not provide a realistic image of natural vulvas."

What's worse is that all too often, the vulvas women see in porn are the only comparison point they have. Compared to boys, girls spend less time exploring their bodies while growing up. Plus, while it's easy for men to sneak a peek at another dude's junk in changing rooms, women have no alternative information for them to realize that the vulvas they see in porn don't represent the entire spectrum of normal.

Fortunately, that same research group from Amsterdam has found a very easy way to counteract the negative effects of porn on our genital body image: simply exposing women to different, unaltered vulvas to show them the full range of normal variation instantly makes them feel better about their own. Women don't want a "designer vagina," they simply want to look normal "down there." So let's find a way to let them know that they already do.

How do our society's body ideals affect you?

"When I was in middle school I was a big fan of Jane Austin and Charles Dickens, whose books were written when tuberculosis was known as 'the romantic disease.' I wished I was frail and pale like the beautiful heroines of the stories, and it wasn't until later that I realized just how dangerous a body ideal that was."

"I am a victim of the '90s heroin chic ideal of beauty. I don't like excess pounds on my body, and I don't think that 'strong is the new skinny.' Most of all, I hate my legs: they are too short, too big, too hairy, too knobby."

"I am generally satisfied with my appearance, but I am well represented in all aspects of media. I am a white, thin, under thirty, able-bodied, cisgendered woman. I really doubt my reserves of self-confidence would be as strong as they are if I didn't see people like myself being validated all the time."

"Once, as a teenager, I was flipping through a magazine and my father overheard me say, 'I wish I looked like the model on the cover.' He replied, 'She wishes she looked like that, too, I bet. Because it's not real.' I have to remember that a lot."

"I am very self-conscious about my weight and especially my middle, because even when I see 'curvy girls' in the media, they always have this smooth silhouette, they are not lumpy. They must be wearing layers of shapewear."

"I hate being small. I'd read articles about how 'real women have curves,' and I'd see comments from other women about how 'nobody wants a stick' and these made me feel even more like I'd never be attractive to a guy because I wasn't enough of a woman. Nobody understands these insecurities, because they all think it's a blessing to be so skinny and small."

Primped, plucked, polished: The business of female grooming standards

If you think our culture's body ideals are unrealistic and discriminatory, brace yourself! Because when it comes to the beauty side of things, our standards are looking even worse. All you need to do is watch any movie from the 1980s to realize that this intense level of groomed perfection that we are so used to seeing—all those perfectly chiseled noses, sparkly white veneers, and baby-smooth complexions—is a very recent development.

These days, looking any less than perfectly groomed comes with major repercussions for women. There are endless examples where women got chastised by both major media outlets and people on social media for minute and completely natural bodily features that, had they been male, no one would have batted an eye over: When record-breaking US gymnast Gabby Douglas had just won her third Olympic medal in Rio de Janeiro, for example, and people went crazy about her hair looking "messy" and "unkempt." When Cardi B performed at the Grammys and was shamed for having a few hairs on her stomach. Or the countless times when a bit of acne on a celebrity's face made the front page of tabloid newspapers.

Considering all of this body policing, it's no wonder women and girls today feel self-conscious about things that used to be complete nonissues just a decade ago and that many are willing to go to extreme lengths to fix or cover up tiny "flaws," like the expression lines on their forehead, the bump on their nose, or a little redness on their cheek. Or that they feel the need to apologize for looking "disgusting" when they haven't had time to do their makeup, or that they warn their significant others about the itty bit of hair on their legs.

How did we ever get to this place?

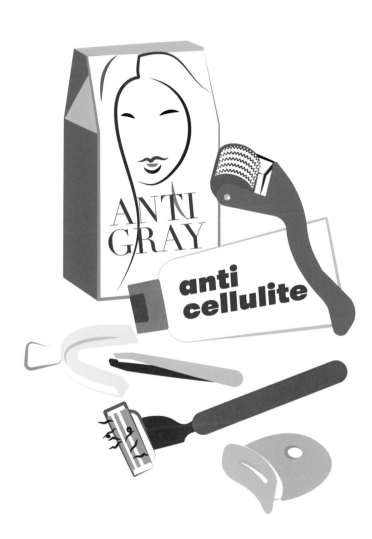

> **"I'm not jealous of my male colleagues often, but I am when it comes to how they can just shower, shave, put on a suit, and be ready to go. The few times I've gone out in public without makeup, it's made the news."**
>
> Hillary Clinton

Why our beauty baseline keeps escalating

Much like fashion, beauty holds a firm spot in mainstream media, and we hear about new products, "innovative" treatments, and the latest trends everywhere: in magazines, commercials, blogs—even high-brow magazines like *The New Yorker* run articles like "Modern Primers for Naturally Glowing Skin" on the regular. This ubiquity of beauty content is problematic because as much as brands and magazine editors would like to have you believe that buying the latest foundation, skin-care gadget, or two-hundred-dollar treatment is an act of empowerment, self-care, or self-expression, the key message underlying the majority of beauty articles and ads is still: this will help you become more attractive.

Now you may be thinking, so what? If beauty products make people feel better about their skin, their hair, or whatever thing they feel insecure about, aren't they helping women's body image? Unfortunately, no, for one crucial reason: beauty companies are not just in the business of selling solutions; they are also in the business of selling *problems.* In fact, many of the "flaws" we want to fix nowadays—and that whole shelves at Sephora are dedicated to—were not considered flaws at all until the beauty industry decided to label them as such.

- Women were not worried about body hair until 1915, when a group of companies selling hair-removal cream invested in a four-year advertising campaign to convince women that smooth underarms were the latest fashionable must-have. Leg hair became a no-go in much the same way twenty years later.

- Women weren't worried about dimply thighs until 1973, when *Vogue* magazine introduced its readers to a fun new thing from France: "Cellulite, the new word for fat you couldn't lose before." As Naomi Wolf states in her book *The Beauty Myth*: "Before 1973, it was normal female flesh."

- Women weren't manicuring their hands until Cutex, the first developer of nail polish and cuticle remover, ran campaigns to convince them that their social standing depended on it: "Embarrassed fingers that shrink from scrutiny—or charming fingers that seek the light!"

- Gray hair wasn't considered a big deal until Clairol told women in the 1940s that their grays were responsible for their nonbustling social life: "Are your friends drifting away from you . . . finding excuses to break appointments . . . failing to call you? That happens so very often to a gray-haired woman . . . sometimes because people think she looks too old to have fun . . . sometimes because they think she looks too old to *be* fun."

All of those new problems didn't replace others but just got added to the long list of body parts women were already worrying about. On top of that comes the fact that just like any other industry, the beauty industry has continuously upped their game and developed new, better products, causing our existing beauty standards to inflate:

- Shiny, white teeth were always on people's wishlists, but it wasn't until the 1990s, when in-office teeth whitening was developed, that white teeth started to literally mean "white-as-snow," and we became unhappy with the natural bone color of our teeth.

- Before Botox hit the scene, fine lines around the forehead and eyes were just normal—actresses and models alike had them. Now, even people in their twenties worry about tiny expression lines and actresses who don't go down the Botox route are considered "brave."

- And you can bet that before dermal fillers exploded in popularity—and you could still find celebrities with non-plumped-up faces on TV—people weren't worrying about their cheeks or their totally normal nasolabial folds or their medium-sized lips.

Of course, it's understandable why beauty companies continue to come out with more and more products. New products create hype and extra sales. However, now we are at a stage where every single body part can be optimized, without ever having to go under the knife. You can get laser treatment to get rid of lines, pores, stretch marks, and freckles. You can get Botox to slim your jaw and lift your eyebrows. You can get fillers injected to make your nose look straighter or your hands look younger. You can get perfect, natural-looking eyebrows microbladed into your skin. You can pay someone to glue tiny extensions to each one of your eyelashes. You can get radio-frequency therapy to get rid of cellulite. You can freeze away that bulge on your lower tummy. You can steam your vagina to . . . I'm not sure what the goal there is actually, but people do it.

It's irrelevant whether or not the average person would ever choose to have all of these procedures done, could afford to, or is even aware that they exist. Because there are enough people that do all of these things (such as celebrities whose career depends in no small part on their appearance), causing our beauty ideals to keep inflating. And at that point it does affect the average person—big time.

> **"We could literally spend our whole lives doing stuff to make ourselves look better, but wouldn't that be a waste of life? I mean, would you rather be lasering off your body hair and getting fillers, or would you rather be learning how to dance salsa or even just binge-watch your favorite TV show? I know what I'd pick."**

The "Ew" factor

After decades of targeted ads, advertisers have managed to label normal bodily features such as body hair, acne, and pores as "dirty" and thus turned female grooming standards into a question of hygiene.

There is no logical reason why hair on a female leg is considered an issue of cleanliness when it isn't on a male leg. And yet, most women (and men too) have completely swallowed the idea that certain natural features, like body hair, are embarrassing, even gross on a female body. This "ew" factor—the shame and worry about potentially being considered repulsive—is what turns grooming standards such as smooth, hair-free legs from optional to never-without. Because if there's one thing that's even less acceptable to be as a woman than unattractive, it's to be "gross."

How do female grooming standards affect you?

"I've felt ultra-self-conscious about my teeth since mov-
ing to the US where EVERYBODY has perfect teeth.
I don't. I never wore braces—where I grew up it just wasn't
done. I would love to wear red lipstick—but whenever
I put it on, I end up removing it because I feel like it just
accentuates my horrible teeth."

"I wish I could just shave 'a couple of times a week' like
my friends, but I am super hairy and have to shave my
whole body every single day, because I have dark hair
literally everywhere. I hate that I am trapped in this hairy
body sometimes."

"My mom was always very concerned about me looking
'sloppy.' Even when I was just at home she would critlcize
me for wearing pajama pants during the day or having
messy hair. I'm almost thirty now, but I still worry about
not looking polished enough and feel weird without
makeup."

"I HATE having to spend all this time on my outfit,
hair, and makeup and would never do it if I weren't so
self-conscious. I would shave my head, forget about
makeup, and wear jeans and a T-shirt all the time."

"I would never go to work without makeup, just because
when I have in the past people actually asked me if I
wanted to go home, because I looked so sick."

"I don't like that even after I have just shaved my underarms, they still are grayish because the roots are still in
there and my skin is pale. I have, in the past, tweezed out
all the hair in my armpits—it takes forever and hurts for
about a day, but it is so nice and smooth afterward."

Who decided women should be hairless anyway?

The history of female hair removal practices perfectly illustrates the arbitrariness of many of our beauty standards. Hair removal has, of course, been practiced for centuries by different cultures for various reasons. But the fact that women today feel the need to remove *all* of their body hair *all of the time*, and feel unkempt with even the teensiest bit of stubble, is very new.

Why you can thanks *Harper's Bazaar* for your hair removal routine

It is safe to say that in the US until the early twentieth century, both sexes left their body hair alone. Hair removal creams were already on the market, but they were meant for removing stray hairs on the face, neck, and chest only.

Then, everything changed in 1915 with an ad in *Harper's Bazaar* that featured a model in a sleeveless dress with her hands above her head and the slogan: "Summer Dress and Modern Dancing combine to make necessary the removal of objectionable hair." According to an article in *The Journal of American Culture*, that ad kicked off a four-year con-certed effort by hair removal brands to expand their market from ladies with the odd chin hair to *all* the ladies.

At first, the ads promoted hairless underarms as a new fashion accessory, with slogans like "The woman of fashion says the underarm must be as smooth as the face" and "The full charm of the Decollete custom is attained when the underarm is perfectly smooth." None of the ads alluded to cleanliness yet—after all, women in the US had spent a good portion of their adult lives feeling perfectly clean *with* hair.

That changed when in the 1920s more people started working in tight spaces, such as offices and factories, and personal hygiene and "not offending your coworkers" became a common concern. Ads began to insinuate that hair-free pits help you feel cleaner and, not long after, female underarm hair was added to the list of "dirty" bodily products like bad breath, sweat, and body odor that "good women" must never be associated with, and removing body hair from your armpits turned from an optional fashion-led choice into a basic grooming essential.

How our legs lost their fuzz license

Female legs stayed hairy for another twenty or so years. Skirts had already been getting shorter, but the majority of women were not bothered by a bit of leg hair underneath their stockings. If they did shave their legs, it was for one particular outfit or event. Then World War II began, pin-up girls were everywhere, and legs became the new object of male admiration. It also got tricky to get a hold of silk and nylon stockings due to wartime rationing.

Advertisers jumped on the opportunity and hit with another ad attack, this time to position hair-free pins as the essential prerequisite for going bare-legged. That idea quickly caught on; soon, not having perfectly smooth legs was seen as being behind the times and matronly. In 1939, *Harper's Bazaar*'s beauty editor wrote: "A word in passing about legs. Ankle socks on the campus are a fine, old institution and all very well, but not on furry legs. If you must wear socks, you owe it to your associates to get into the habit of using some safe, dependable depilatory. And we mean regularly—not just once in a blue moon as a kind of isolated experiment."

In loving memory of the bush

Alongside pin-up culture, the bikini also gained popularity and, it is likely that as leg hair removal became compulsory, women would also remove any pubic hair that was out-side of the bikini line. But the rest was allowed to stay fully natural—for a while.

In pre-1980s porn, the majority of actresses sported their natural hair. People call it a 1970s bush nowadays, because that's the decade when the first big porn movies started showing explicit shots of vulvas, but really the full au naturel bush is not unique to the 1970s, but to the entire time before that, too.

In the 1980s, porn turned into a huge industry with major budgets and better cameras, which made hair removal a simple question of cinematography: where there is less hair, you can see more.

According to most sources, though, women in real life were trimming and grooming their pubic hair into landing strips or triangles, but not yet baring it all. The full everything-off look did not go mainstream until the turn of the century, when several high-profile celeb-rities touted the life-changing powers of the Brazilian wax. A *Sex and the City* episode in which Carrie gets her pubes professionally ripped out firmly established the "Hollywood cut" as the go-to choice of the independent, stylish, twenty-first-century woman.

Since then, we've promoted the totally bare look from "forward choice" to "default grooming standard." According to a large-scale study from the University of California, 62 percent of women between the ages of eighteen and sixty-five remove all of their pubic hair and only 16 percent go au naturel. Author Peggy Orenstein, who has inter-viewed dozens of young women about the topic for her

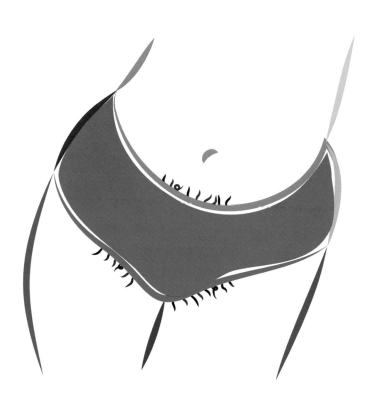

book *Girls & Sex*, believes that although most say they do it for their own satisfaction or hygiene, the real reason so many women remove their pubic hair is simple: shame. We have fully accepted that hair "down there" is embarrassing.

The impact of Eurocentric beauty standards

Our society's beauty ideals are bad news for every woman's self-esteem, but women of color undoubtedly carry a heavier burden because—despite the fact that around four out of ten Americans do not identify as white—our beauty standard is still *Eurocentric*.

The media is still full of subtle and not-so-subtle messages telling women of color that the more Caucasian you look, the better. The vast majority of women who represent beauty in ads and magazine spreads, on TV screens and catwalks, are white. Except for a few rare exceptions, nonwhite women who are admired for their beauty are the ones whose features are closer to the Caucasian "ideal," with lighter skin, a narrower nose, or straighter hair. Natural, textured hair is rarely seen in the media.

The heartbreaking 2005 documentary *A Girl Like Me* by Kiri Davis showed the extent to which even young kids today have still internalized the idea that white equals good. In the film, we see a repeat of the famous doll experiments from 1940: African-American children of preschool age were given the option to choose between two dolls that were exactly the same—except one was white and one was black. Just like in 1940, the majority of the children in Davis's experiment chose the white doll, and they also picked it when asked which doll was nicer or prettier.

"For African-American women, hair is political."

Kathy Russell-Cole, Midge Willson, and Ronald E. Hall, *The Color Complex*

It's never "just hair"

A Girl Like Me also features snippets of young women talking about hair. "You have to have permed hair or relaxed hair. If it's natural, that's even better—that's good hair. Bad hair is hair that you have to relax because it's kinky," says seventeen-year-old Stephanie.

According to writer Cheryl Thompson, the whole "black hair issue" is so complex because hair is a question of identity. "For young black girls, hair is not just something to play with, it is something that is laden with messages, and it has the power to dictate how others treat you, and in turn, how you feel about yourself."

"Historically, the relationship between African-American women and their hair goes back to the days of slavery and is connected with the notion of the color caste system: the belief that the lighter one's skin color, the better one is and that straighter hair is better than kinky hair," writes Tracey Owens Patton, director of African American & Diaspora studies at the University of Wyoming. Those beliefs outlasted the American Civil War and for black people in the twentieth century, with racial segregation still deeply entrenched in every corner of American culture, their hair was a question of respectability, and therefore also of employability.

Straightening soon became the norm, first using temporary methods (such as hair pressing with pomade and a hot comb), then using chemical relaxers, which became commercially available in the 1960s. "Today, it is estimated that 70 to 80 percent of black women chemically straighten their hair," writes Cheryl Thompson. "When you consider that for the past one hundred years manufacturers have almost exclusively only promoted the idea that natural black hair needs to be altered, it all begins to make sense. When was the last time short, curly, kinky black hair was celebrated or promoted as equally as beautiful?"

But in recent years, the natural hair movement, originally kicked off in the 1960s, has gained a second wind and more women are embracing their natural hair, free of relaxers or weaves. In an interview with *Allure* magazine, actress Lupita Nyong'o said: "The upkeep of relaxed hair is a commitment. It took styling it once a week and then having it retouched once a month. I remember doing crazy things, like sleeping with my head above the headboard so that my curls wouldn't get messed up for the next day. I'd have these terrible neckaches because I was determined to keep my hair as pristine as possible. And it was super expensive." And author Chimamanda Ngozi Adichie writes in her novel *Americanah*: "Relaxing your hair is like being in prison. You're caged in. Your hair rules you. You didn't go running with Curt today because you don't want to sweat out this straightness. You're always battling to make your hair do what it wasn't meant to do."

However, some people have also criticized the natural hair movement, observing that many of the women who are being celebrated on social media for wearing their natural hair have looser curls and are often lighter skinned. In an article for *Dazed*, Georgina Lawton writes, "The more African in you and your hair, the less likely you are to see your representation online, with many black women arguing that they are being erased from the movement entirely."

Georgina Lawton notes how, ironically, the popularity of "a movement that preaches inclusivity" is making some women feel shamed for wearing weaves or getting their hair relaxed: "Some of these same naturals also make a smug link between having curly hair and being enlightened, or 'curly conscious.' But, of course, there is no higher purpose to having a looser curl pattern and rocking a 'fro doesn't make you a better feminist or advocate for minority rights—it just means you've exercised a personal choice over your hairstyle."

"Fair & Lovely": Colorism in the 21st century

The global market for skin-whitening products has boomed in recent years. According to a report from Global Industry Analysts, the market was worth $10 billion in 2015 and is expected to reach $31.2 billion by 2024. Skin-lightening products are especially popular in India, Pakistan, the Caribbean, West Africa, and the Asia-Pacific region. According to some estimates, 70 percent of women in West African countries, such as Ghana and Nigeria, use them regularly; almost one-third of Indian women use skin-lightening products every day.

The ads for these types of products—whose active ingredients (mercury and hydroquinone) have been linked to everything from skin cancer to birth defects—often feature pretty blatant appraisals that lighter skin leads to success, love, and happiness, starting with the product names. The most popular product in India, where more than $400 million of skin-whitening products are sold each year, is called Fair & Lovely (the version for men is called Fair & Handsome). In an article for *Business of Fashion*, Maliha Rehman writes, "The adverts for the cream tend to follow a staid format, where a dark-skinned girl is unable to get a job or get married until she uses the product and manages to lighten her skin."

People are quick to point to the globalization of Western pop culture as the driving factor behind the boom of lightening products. But in many parts of the world, lighter skin has been associated with a higher social status for centuries. Maliha Rehman writes, "Beauty regimes that celebrate light skin are ancient and varied. In Pakistan and India, girls are told to 'drink less tea and more milk' for whiter skin and a healthy brown tan is studiously avoided. An old African adage cautions that fair-skinned women are more expensive to marry. In Japan, an ancient proverb dictates that 'white skin covers the seven flaws,' implying that even if a woman's features are not attractive, her fair skin can make up for it."

According to *The Color Complex: The Politics of Skin Color in a New Millennium* by Karen Russell-Cole, Midge Wilson, and Ronald E. Hall, "Among many adult Indian women, memories of mothers warning them to get out of the sun remain vivid. The harsh reality, according to Indian parents, is that it is simply harder to marry off a darker-skinned daughter, especially if she is poor. So worried do some parents get about a daughter's dark skin ruining her chances for matrimony that they are willing to spend what little family money there is to buy skin lighteners for her to apply."

But things are changing—slowly. In India and many other parts of the world where skin whitening is popular, there have been campaigns to end the stigma around darker skin. In the US, magazines face intense backlash for lightening the complexions of their models. And after years of exclusively offering shades of beige, more and more makeup companies are making the long-overdue effort to have their foundations, concealers, and other products work for the full spectrum of skin colors.

"But attitudes toward ancient beauty standards that have been exacerbated by centuries of colonialism and a global fashion and beauty industry perpetuating Eurocentric beauty ideals are slow to change," says Rehman. "It will take many more campaigns and movements for the obsession around lighter skin to dim."

Ageism: The grim saga of "younger is better"

When I was writing this book, three of my closest friends all had their thirtieth birthdays coming up, and the rest of our friend group was talking about how we should celebrate. Our plans to throw them a big hello-thirty bash were quickly shot down by the birthday girls themselves: "Why would I want to celebrate the fact that I'll be officially old? No thank you." Of course, we'd heard it all before. Just like we're used to complaining about the weather, stress, and politicians, complaining about your age is now a totally acceptable thing to do—whether you're twenty, forty, or eighty years old. The trouble is that unlike complaining about the weather, complaining about your age is not just empty rhetoric; it reflects the very real fear women have of growing—and looking—older.

That fear is reflected in our day-to-day habits, with women spending a fortune on antiaging skin-care products, Botox being used on people in their early twenties, and our collective sunscreen obsession. One woman told me, "I try to avoid being in direct sunlight, and unless it's the dead of winter I make sure to reapply my sunscreen at least every three hours. It can be a bit exhausting at times, but I just really don't want to get wrinkles." Another woman I talked to told me that in order to prevent wrinkles she had trained herself to not frown or squint her eyes—ever.

"I hate aging and am struggling with it, but I feel like growing old gracefully is more attractive, so bizarrely, vanity is what has propelled me into not doing too much to combat it."

The fear is real—and understandable. In our culture, messages that "old equals unattractive" are everywhere. A huge chunk of the beauty industry is centered around framing lines and wrinkles—natural by-products of being alive—as the enemy, to sell products. Women who "age well" are celebrated and admired in magazines and on TV as if it were a form of achievement. In fact, it is not helpful at all when people point to someone like Halle Berry or Julianne Moore as evidence that women over a "certain" age can be attractive, too, because it does nothing but highlight—once again—that in order to be beautiful you have to look young for your age. If we ever get to a point where we consider a female face that is full of lines beautiful and desirable, then we've really gotten somewhere.

Why we need a female James Bond

When it comes to age, the level of diversity we see on TV and in movies is in the same dire state as it is for body shapes and ethnicities. Practically all models and actresses in big box office hits are in their twenties or thirties, or sometimes their early forties—as long as they *look* like a twenty-something, of course.

But the problems with age representation in our culture goes far beyond discriminatory casting choices. Because not only do we rarely see actresses over thirty-five star in major movie roles, but we are also barely exposed to stories of women over thirty-five at all, no matter the medium!

"Youth and beauty are not accomplishments, they're the temporary happy by-products of time and/or DNA. Don't hold your breath for either."

Carrie Fisher

How many movies, TV shows, even books, can you think of with female characters over forty who lead full lives, have ambitions, have love interests? There are *plenty* of men aged forty, fifty, and sixty who do cool stuff in movies, but badass female characters over forty? Few and far between.

When you take into account this epic lack of stories, it's really no big shocker that we've reached a point where even young women dread their next birthday. Our fear of *looking* older is all jumbled up with a general fear of *being* older, which is exacerbated by the fact that as women we've been told all our lives that our youth is the only time that really matters, the only time we get to do fun stuff and experience the world. Time is running out.

"I have so much respect for older women, and I know there are amazing aspects to all ages in life, so I'm just along for the fun of the ride!"

Ashton Applewhite, author of *This Chair Rocks: A Manifesto against Ageism,* believes that if we want to combat our fear of aging, we need to stop looking to the media for role models. "What we need is to literally come together, make friends of all ages, and talk about how we feel. If younger women can look past the 'She has wrinkles, I don't want to be like her' bias that we've all internalized from a lifetime of being brainwashed by the media, and actually talk to older women, they will tell you that they love being the age they are, and how aging brings confidence and clarity. As a younger woman you can be like, "'Guess what? I'm going to age into this power, and this sense of self-knowledge.'"

How do you feel about the prospects of growing and looking older?

"It seems like signs of aging are becoming as much of a no-no as being fat. If you look old, it means you've been lazy. You've lacked discipline, you have bad genes, or—worst of all—you've given up."

"I've been using eye cream since I was a teen. I'm thinking about getting into face yoga and I have also considered Botox or face acupuncture for the lines between my brows."

"I'm worried that I won't be able to accept the changes my body will go through when I age, because I had a really hard time accepting the cellulite that I got in my early twenties. I hope that by then I will have cultivated a more relaxed attitude."

"I have been seriously, dangerously ill. That shook my world upside down. Being healthy now has more meaning than ever, and growing old is something I look forward to, instead of being scared of."

"I am not afraid of wrinkles, but I am afraid of getting the wrong kind of wrinkles. I don't want frown lines. I feel like smile wrinkles will show a life well lived whereas frown lines will show a life that was filled with sorrow and stress."

"I'm sad about growing and looking older. Seems I've only just begun to make peace with how I look, and now it's all changing for the worse."

"I hope I get to grow a lot older! My parents died in their early seventies, so I spend a lot more time worrying about dying young than worrying about looking old."

"I'm twenty-seven and already doing a full antiaging routine. I'm terrified of looking older; I wear sunscreen every day and make sure to reapply throughout the day."

"I feel a bit of apprehension about growing and looking older, but I am surrounded by quite a few older and aging women of grace, humor, and—yes—beauty! I hope to follow their example."

"I have a lot of anxiety about aging! I worry that I will lose a source of power if I'm not attractive. It's stupid because I'd feel terrible to learn that people were only treating me a certain way because they thought I looked hot, and yet at the same time, it feels like this security blanket."

CHAPTER 6

MORE THAN A BODY

Feeling good about yourself is a basic human need. We all have an internal self-worth barometer that's constantly being fed with new information from our brain and recalibrating exactly how good we feel about ourselves at any given moment. Your boss compliments your performance? The needle jumps up. You see a bad photo of yourself on social media? The needle goes down. Totally normal.

The problem is that many women's self-worth barometer is buggy. After years of being bombarded with societal messages about the importance of beauty, our self-worth barometers have started to overvalue one factor: our appearance. For many of us, how we feel about the way we look has become the deciding factor for how we feel about ourselves, our worth as a person, our life, everything. When we think we look good, we have confidence for days, but when we think we look bad, we feel defeated, and none of our other accomplishments matter.

If you have a sneaky feeling your own self-worth barometer may depend a little too much on the way you look, it's not enough to just push B-E-A-U-T-Y off its pedestal. You also need to replace it with something. You need to understand—on both a conscious and a visceral level—that you are worthy for a whole lot of reasons other than your appearance.

What's wrong with deriving confidence from the way you look?

In our culture, encouraging women to derive confidence through the way they look is a pretty routine thing. Everything from makeup to shapewear to breast implants is marketed as "confidence-boosting" these days. Fitness influencers teach us "Twelve Easy Moves for More Body Confidence this Summer." Beauty brands sell "Confidence in a Cleanser." And you too may be thinking: "I often like the way I look or at least parts of it and now you want to take that away from me, too?"

But don't worry: it's totally A-okay to derive short-term confidence boosts from the way you look. Nobody is saying you shouldn't feel good about a new haircut, or looking great in a dress, or whatever. It's normal that how we feel about our body makes up some portion of our self-esteem. But you definitely want to avoid basing your whole self-esteem on your looks for one simple reason: it's one hell of a risky business!

Your body is a living thing, and it will change over the course of your life—whether through aging, pregnancy, an illness, an accident, weight loss, weight gain, or a new physical hobby. And considering how volatile our beauty ideals have been thus far, it's very likely that they will change in your lifetime, too. Who knows, maybe the next big thing will be Hulk Hogan—sized quads and here you've been feeling so great about your dainty little pins. Just because you fit the beauty standard right now does not mean you'll still fit it in five years.

If you have always relied on feeling attractive to feel good about yourself as a person, a tiny beauty disruption like a ten-pound weight gain, a sudden bout of acne, or a scar from necessary surgery can pull the rug out from under you. Something as external and unstable as beauty is a terrible foundation to build your self-worth on.

So, in short: it's totally fine to care about what you look like and derive some self-esteem from it; just make sure you know you have plenty of other stuff to offer as well.

**BEYOND
BEAUTIFUL
TOOLBOX**

The Beyond Beautiful portfolio

Just because your self-worth barometer is concentrating a little too hard on appearances at the moment doesn't mean you don't already know that you have strengths and qualities outside of the way you look. After a lifetime of living in a looks-obsessed society, those thoughts—all of your positive memories and feelings of accomplishment—just got pushed to the back of your mind. But now it's time to dust them off. Remind yourself of all the reasons you kick ass, all the reasons you're beyond beautiful.

Step 1: List your positive qualities

Start with a good old-fashioned brainstorm:

- What positive qualities do you have?

- What skills, talents, or strengths do you have?

- What achievements (big or small) are you most proud of?

- What challenges have you overcome?

- What are you grateful for?

If you find it difficult to come up with these, try shifting your perspective a little:

- How would you answer these questions in your happiest, most confident moments?

- How would the people in your life that you are closest to describe you?

- Which qualities or skills that you admire in others do you also possess?

Step 2: Find concrete examples and reminisce

Once you have a list full of qualities and strengths, select five to fifteen items that feel the most significant to you. Then, on a new page, describe at least one (but ideally more) concrete example or situation where you showed each quality or strength in detail. Feel free to expand your list whenever you feel like it, and add more examples as they happen.

Step 3: Keep reminding yourself

Keep your Beyond Beauty portfolio close by so any time your judgy inner voice is acting up or you are having a low-confidence moment, you can pull it out and remind yourself of the many ways that you are worthy and wonderful.

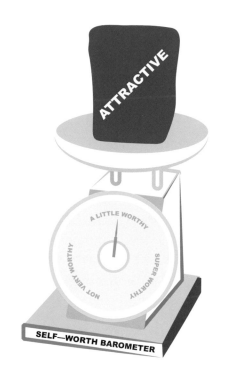

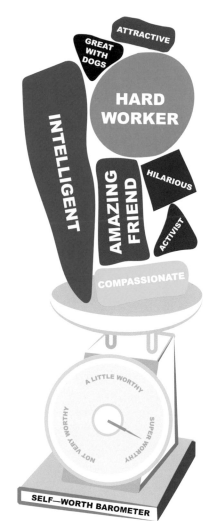

Moving in today: Your positive inner voice

Remember your uber-judgy inner voice? Well, it is about to meet its match. Because now that you've built up your Beyond Beautiful portfolio, you are ready to start working on one of the most important techniques when it comes to beating body insecurities or any other type of self-esteem issues: your *positive* inner voice.

How does it work? Easy: from now on, whenever you demonstrate one of the qualities from your portfolio, acknowledge it. For example, let's say you're once again putting in extra hours at the office to make sure your pitch for the next day is as good as it can be. For a brief moment, pause and give yourself the recognition you deserve: "I'm a hard worker; I can persevere."

If that seems a little weird or exhausting, remember: you are already commenting on yourself *negatively* all the time. What you are trying to do is to simply be a little fairer to yourself by paying equal attention to your good traits when you exhibit them.

As with so many things, in the beginning you'll have to actively push yourself to do this. But eventually, those happy, appreciative thoughts will simply pop into your head, and your new positive voice will have lodged itself into your brain and help you collect plenty of evidence that you're actually a pretty great, worthy, and lovable person—regardless of how you look on the outside.

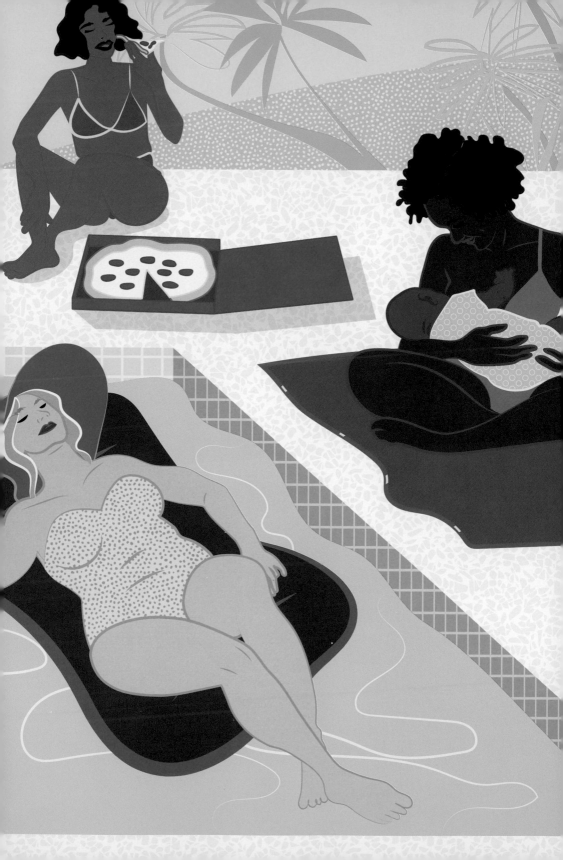

PART III

TAKE BACK
THE POWER

CHAPTER 7

I CAN'T TONIGHT, I FEEL FAT

You know how you can tell when someone has a great body image? When they think that having a bad body image is no big deal. "So what, you know you're no beauty queen, who cares? Talk about first-world problems . . . "

But body image *is* a big deal, because it's a question of freedom. Yes, a lack of confidence affects what you see in the mirror, but what's way worse is that it convinces you that you *can't do things* because of the way your body looks—wearing shorts, for example, or going out without makeup that covers your acne, or dancing, or speaking in front of a big crowd. And so you wear long pants even during summer, apply layers of foundation and concealer every single morning, watch your friends' drinks while they hit the dance floor, and turn down invitations to events, even when they'd mean a big career opportunity for you. You are no longer in the driver's seat of your own life; your body image is calling the shots for you.

Many of the women I spoke to have adopted something of a "just do it" approach to deal with their urge to hide or run, where they've perfected the art of white-knuckling their way through a pool party, gym class, or presentation. And yeah, that can work. But wouldn't it be great if a day at the pool didn't require a bucket full of willpower to get through, and you could just enjoy your time, perhaps even look forward to it?

So you're afraid of being judged

Although flinging yourself in front of whatever you're scared of can work, a much gentler approach to get over your tendency to run or hide is to understand that the thing you're afraid of isn't a threat in the first place. So let's take a closer look at exactly what is going on in your head when you are about to decline an invitation or otherwise choose *not* to do something because of the way your body looks.

I have flaws that warrant some kind of shame.
↓
If I expose my flaws others will judge me.
↓
I will feel terrible.

The typical (subconscious) thought process underlying avoidance behaviors consists of a three-level chain of assumptions that we, of course, treat as facts when we are in the middle of it all. Your judgy inner voice is hard at work, whispering to you all the terrible things that are definitely going to happen, should you decide to move off that towel. If you want to not only move off the towel but also feel good about it, you need to poke holes in your judgy inner voice's logic. Tackle each assumption one by one to convince it and yourself that you will be okay.

Assumption 1: I have flaws that warrant some form of shame

Shame is the basis for pretty much all of the negative stuff we think, feel, and do in relation to our bodies, which is why we spent several earlier chapters of this book putting our society's beauty ideals in perspective. Remind your judgy inner voice of what you've learned.

Are there activities you avoid because you feel insecure about your looks?

"I have stopped dancing in studios because dance is an expression of the whole body and if you are not confident, it is just too difficult to perform in front of people."

"I don't go swimming. Ever. Even on holiday with my kids. My husband goes in the sea with them and I wade in the shallows. I have my camera, taking photos of them all as an excuse for why I'm not in with them."

"One day, when I was traveling around South America with friends, we came across this amazing waterfall. We hadn't brought swimming gear, so my friends just stripped to their underwear to go swim under the waterfall. I stayed on the edge and watched. There was no way I was stripping to my underwear and letting everyone see my horrible body. I really regret that now."

"If I have pimples, I won't go out. I'll straight up bail on an event, cancel last minute, etc. When I have pimples and my makeup is all caked on and super noticeable, I can't focus on anything but that. I can see the people I'm talking to looking at it, and it makes me feel so insecure."

"Sometimes I might feel wary about going to the beach or doing sports with others (tight-clothes kind of sports), but then I remind myself that others are not perfect either, so I will be okay. For the first few moments I might feel awkward, but later on I usually relax and enjoy whatever it is I am doing."

"I often avoid sex, and when I do have sex, it's hard for me to stop thinking about rolls on my stomach or faces I'm making. I can almost never give myself over to the bodily experience of it."

YOU ARE NOT ALONE

No matter what it is that you are ashamed of, whether it is your weight, cellulite, or so on, remember that it is a natural aspect of the human body in all of its facets that millions of other women worldwide share with you. Some of them may feel like you do, but then others are completely fine with it.

IT'S NOT YOU, IT'S THEM

The way you look is not the reason you feel ashamed—it is because you were taught by a bad system. The fact that we feel shame for things that are inherently natural makes no logical sense and is entirely culturally constructed.

Assumption 2: If I expose my flaws others will judge me

Really, we could stop right here. Your flaws don't warrant shame, that's it— have fun at the beach! But just for funsies, let's move on and think about the second assumption your judgy inner voice is making: that once you expose your "flaw," others will move their opinion of you down a notch.

WOULD YOU JUDGE OTHERS FOR THIS?

If you saw a woman with cellulite or a scar or whatever you are worried about, would you think of her in the way that you are afraid of being thought of? Or would you simply think, "There is a woman who has a scar," and make no further judgment because you are a grown-up with morals and manners?

WOULD THE PEOPLE IN YOUR LIFE THAT YOU RESPECT JUDGE OTHERS FOR THIS?

Think about some of the people in your life whose opinion is important to you. Your friends, your relatives, perhaps your coworkers or boss: would they judge other women for having the specific physical aspect you feel self-conscious about?

DOES THE OPINION OF PEOPLE WHO WOULD JUDGE OTHERS MATTER TO YOU?

Sure, there are shitty people in this world who, for one reason or another, believe in superficial stereotypes. But does the opinion of those people matter to you? No. It has no effect on your life.

Assumption 3: I will feel terrible

"But what if they do judge you," your judgy inner voice may now be saying. "What if they look at you in this specific way that makes it super obvious they're thinking you're too fat to be wearing a bikini? You would feel awful for the rest of the week; it's just too risky."

If your inner voice believes that one judgy look or snarky comment is going to send you into a huge downward spiral, remind it that you've already lived through a lot. As a woman in this world, you're confronted with body-shaming, body policing, and sexism from other people and the media all the time. And even when something hurt you on a deeper level, you got over it, and you're here now. You are more resilient than you give yourself credit for. So even if shit hits the fan (although it most definitely won't), you can deal!

What would Serena do? (Or, why you need a confidence role model)

If you're struggling to get over your fears of potential and seemingly life-threatening judgment, try this shortcut: put yourself in the shoes of someone else! Someone who possesses that same feature you feel insecure about and whom you admire for their confidence and general badass-ery— whether it's someone you know in real life, a celebrity, or even a fictional character.

Pick your confidence role model and then whenever you are in a situation where you're about to cancel, decline, or decide against some activity because of body-image worries, ask yourself: What would Serena Williams do? Or Tiffany Haddish? Or Arya Stark? Or Ruth Bader Ginsberg? Would she feel self-conscious in your situation? What would her advice to you be?

Step #4
Wiggle your bits front and center

Step #3
Join the dance class but stay in the back

Step #2
Take a short stretching class

Step #1
Walk on the treadmill and take a look around

**BEYOND
BEAUTIFUL
TOOLBOX**

The confidence ladder: How to get over any fear step-by-step

Once you have questioned your own logic, you are ready to face your fears—but in a gradual way. You don't want to jump right into the deep end and get overwhelmed again. Instead, dip your toes into the water first, so you can see that nothing bad is happening. Then, go a little further, until you feel comfortable to go all the way.

Before you start, you need a plan. Psychologists call this a "ladder of success" or "confidence ladder": a list of gradually harder activities that you can face one by one. You can use confidence ladders to overcome any type of avoidance habit, whether it's the running or hiding kind.

Want an example? Okay, let's say you would love to take that cardio dance class at your local gym but have always felt self-conscious about exercising in public and the thought of letting loose in front of everyone feels insurmountable. Instead of immediately giving up on your idea, you could start with a baby step in the right direction and go to the gym to simply walk on the treadmill and take a look around. Do this as often as you need to until you feel comfortable enough to climb step two: taking a stretching class. Then, when the gym no longer feels such a scary and judgmental place, you'll perhaps be brave enough to actually join a dance class, even just for a couple of minutes. And who knows, perhaps in a couple of weeks, you'll be wiggling your bits front and center.

You get the idea: The last step of your ladder is your goal behavior, and your starting step should be something you can see yourself accomplishing without too much effort. Each next stage should only feel a little harder than the one before. It's up to you how many steps you include. If you need ten, then go ahead and use ten.

Always tackle new steps when you are in a generally good frame of mind. Don't try to cram it in after a frustrating day at work or when you feel hungry, tired, anxious, or otherwise grumpy. And if you set out to climb a step one day and it doesn't work, don't beat yourself up about it. Just try again next time!

"Ironically, practicing ballet—standing in front of a mirror and gaping at myself for hours on end— is what it took for me to finally get comfortable in my own body."

Don't make me look: When you're avoiding mirrors and cameras

Sometimes we run or hide not because we fear the judgment of others, but because we ourselves don't want to be confronted with how we look. When we consciously look at the floor every time we walk past a mirror or refuse to click on a photo we got tagged in, there is no one there to judge us but ourselves, but that doesn't mean the judgment isn't just as painful, perhaps even more so. We know that hits to our self-esteem hurt and that they make everything else in our life harder, so we try to protect ourselves as best as we can.

Regardless of whether you are worried about your own or other people's judgment, the steps to overcoming an avoidance habit are the same: question your logic, then face your fears by climbing your way to the top of a confidence ladder. So look at yourself! Do it until your own reflection is no longer the scary monster you've made it out to be. Then move on with your life.

I have flaws that warrant some kind of shame.

↓

If I expose my flaws others will judge me. *I* *myself*

↓

I will feel terrible.

CHAPTER 8

SOCIAL MEDIA

Social media no doubt influences our lives in many positive ways: it brings us together, gives everyone a voice, and allows us to find people who think and feel like us. From a body-image perspective, though, social media is kind of a mixed bag. Yes, it has been a huge driver of the movement toward female empowerment and more diversity in the media. At the same time, studies show that many aspects of social media can also be pretty bad news for body image.

But don't worry: I'm not going to tell you to swear off Instagram, quit your selfie habit, or delete your Facebook account. But if you suspect your social media use may be putting a damper on your body image, it pays to take a closer look at exactly what you're doing online, and how it affects you, both as a consumer and as a producer of social media content. And then feel free to cherry-pick!

The real reason your feeds put you in a funk

Let's talk about media literacy. Most people are media literate when it comes to movies, ad campaigns, and magazines: they know that those images don't represent reality and that plenty of behind-the-scenes tricks and Photoshop were involved to create them. Studies have shown that this media literacy is one of the most powerful antidotes to low body confidence, because if you know that something isn't real, you're not going to compare yourself to it. The problem is that even though media literacy for movies and magazines is at an all-time high, women are still much less likely to view pics they see on Instagram, Facebook, and other social sites with the same critical eye, for one reason: social media images give off the illusion of being unedited, candid shots of real life.

That faux candidness is what makes social media—more than any other type of media—such a minefield for our self-esteem. We have always admired movie stars and models for the way they looked. But thanks to social media, there is no longer a clear line between "normal" and "paid-to-look-this good-with-a-glam-squad-on-the-payroll." When you see a red carpet, magazine cover, or movie screen, it's easy to imagine how much work must have gone into creating that image. Now we see those same celebrities on their days off and without makeup, looking every bit as gorgeous. We also see a whole bunch of other people—influencers—who may earn a living by looking the way they do, but who are supposed to be regular folks just like us, giving us a candid glimpse into their everyday life.

"Social media gives us a snapshot of everyone else's best days. No one posts about the days when they didn't have time to do their hair and could only find their old clumpy mascara."

The trouble is, of course, that much—no, scratch that—the *majority* of what you see on social media is anything but candid and everyday. There are filters, lighting tricks, and Photoshop. We've all heard stories of the burned-out social media starlet who confessed to regularly taking more than a hundred photos for a single Instagram post, always on an empty stomach and as dehydrated as possible, to bring out her abs. If someone's social media account is (part of) their business, you can be damn sure that they are approaching it like one: they plan, they test, they optimize—just like any other business would. And that's their prerogative. As long as you, on the receiving end, are aware that this influencer's selfie and that brand's Insta story are not simple snapshots of reality but staged images with a clear (and often commercial) purpose, it's all good. Because then you also know that it makes zero sense to compare yourself to them.

The problem with social media is not that it's full of gorgeous, successful, stylish people. It's that it's full of gorgeous, successful, stylish people who are supposed to be *just like us*. We are mistaking center stage during show time for off-season behind the scenes. Social media is a stage—one that anyone can hop on and do their bit—but a stage nonetheless.

REFLECTION QUESTIONS

What effect do you believe social media has on your body image?

Do you sometimes feel envious, jealous, or inadequate because of social media? If so, what type of images trigger those feelings the most?

To what extent do you believe images on social media are edited and/or staged?

Selfies: Empowering or problematic?

A thousand selfies are uploaded to Instagram every ten seconds, and every third photo taken by a millennial is a selfie. Clearly, we're obsessed. And it's not hard to see why. Selfies are perhaps the easiest, most direct way to express your mood, your personality, your opinion. They help you document your life, get creative, take a stance, and discover, build, and share your own personal brand. But, unfortunately, it's not all rosy in selfie-land. Because when it comes to our body image, a selfie habit can put you in the danger zone, for two reasons.

Are you selfie-objectifying?

If we took our selfies with the same point-shoot-check-done approach that we use to take other pictures, it would all be fine. But, of course, the typical selfie routine is a lot more elaborate than that: many women told me about taking tens, sometimes hundreds, of pictures from marginally different angles and with varying lighting, poses, and facial expressions—all for a single selfie.

After the shooting comes the selection process where all those photos need to be scrutinized and ranked, until the "most flattering shot" can be crowned. When we do all this, when we examine our face and body from a purely aesthetic perspective, carefully gauging how others will see us, we're not just nitpicking ourselves to the ground, we're also engaging in perhaps the purest form of self-objectification there is. Lindsay and Lexie Kite call it *selfie-objectification*: "[Selfies] are a clear reflection of exactly what girls and women have been taught to be their entire lives: images to be looked at. Carefully posed, styled, and edited images of otherwise dynamic human beings for others to gaze upon and comment on."

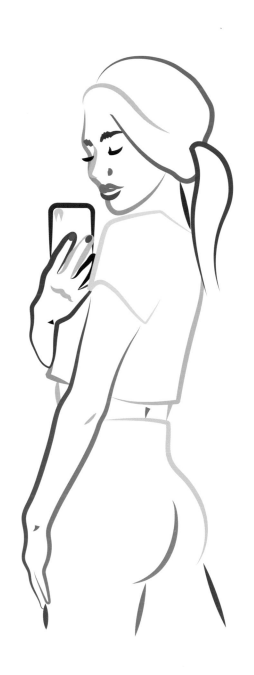

You vs. your fantasy self

Social media is a public place, so it's only natural that we want to put our best foot forward, especially when it comes to selfies, and technology has provided us with a lot of options to do just that, from filters to Facetune. However, psychologist Renee Engeln found that it's exactly this ability to create fantasy versions of ourselves that so often has a very negative effect on our body image. In her book *Beauty Sick*, she writes, "You have more control over your appearance online than you do in the real world. You can cull the best photo from hundreds taken. You can choose lighting and poses designed to flatter. You can filter. You can use Photoshop. But the more you see a version of yourself that doesn't really exist, the more foreign the woman in the mirror will feel to you and the less satisfied you'll become with her."

"I got good at using Photoshop in middle school and have always edited pretty much any picture that goes on social media. The photos still look like me, and friends don't usually believe that they're edited unless I show them my process, so I always tell myself that I'm just terribly unphotogenic and look better in real life."

The conclusion here is easy: selfie away, but hold the fussing. Remind yourself of the purpose behind your selfie: are you trying to prove to everyone how hot you are, or are you trying to capture a great moment and express yourself? Unless it's the former, resist the urge to perfect your angles, perfect your pose, or perfect your complexion. Because what good is a perfect social media feed when your body image is down in the dumps?

**BEYOND
BEAUTIFUL
TOOLBOX**

How to stop feeling Instagram-inadequate

If you are on social media, you're probably no stranger to that sinking feeling in your gut when you scroll past yet another moonlit-vacation pic of a photogenic human being who seems to have all the things you want in life, including a cute dog, a sexy millionaire lover, and a successful career. Feeling Instragram-inadequate is neither fun nor productive, so the next time you see a potential "Oh my god, why don't I look/live/am like her" trigger, try this strategy: instead of delving straight into in-depth comparison mode, pretend you are a researcher who's interested in social media culture. Investigate five aspects:

1. **Purpose.** Why did this account or this person decide to post this photo? What response are they hoping for?

2. **Message.** What is the overt message of this photo (for example: "I feel so lucky to be able to witness this beautiful sunset #blessed")? What is the subliminal message ("I can afford expensive vacations")?

3. **Production.** Who took the photo? Is the person in it lost in thoughts or is she concentrating on holding what looks like a pretty uncomfortable pose? Where was the shot taken? Does the scene look real or carefully arranged? What about the lighting and editing?

4. **Meaning.** Based on the picture, what can you really infer about this person and her life? Does the shot of this gorgeous lady with ripped abs and capped shoulders mean her life is nothing but sunshine and rainbows? Or does it simply mean she spends a lot of time in the gym and knows how to pose, but probably still goes through the same ups and downs as everyone else?

5. **Relevance.** Social media tricks aside, the reality is that there will always be people who have what you want, whether that is confidence, an amazing career, a loving relationship, whatever. But does their attainment in that one area take away from your ability to be happy and successful and reach your goals as well? Nope. It has zero relevance.

How does social media affect your body image?

"I think social media can be beneficial for women's body image, because it gives us a chance to see a much wider variety of body shapes and types. Before, with traditional mass media, we had no control over what types of bodies we are shown. On social media, the most popular influencers may have stereotypical body types too, but at least you are able to unfollow them and instead follow accounts that show more diverse body shapes."

"Social media—and in particular the body positive and disability communities—has opened up a whole new world for me. As a wheelchair-bound, overweight woman with nontraditional features, I used to feel resigned to a life of feeling inadequate, but seeing all those strong, powerful women on social media living their best lives has given me so much confidence."

"Social media certainly works against women over forty-five. Influencers are young and, if not, then blessed with slim bodies and ageless beauty. Only ex-models get to speak for women over forty-five, which makes it pretty irrelevant."

"Social media liberated me. I don't post pictures of myself for the sake of counting likes and collecting compliments. I share sweet moments that are worth remembering. I follow people who have beautiful minds and have something important to say. I really think how we use social media matters."

"When I was growing up, I could avoid advertisements by muting commercials or not picking up fashion magazines. Now, those advertisements are intermixed with the truly 'social' aspect of social media, the part that offers friendship and connection, making them much harder to ignore."

"I created an Instagram account to share landscape photographs I take while hiking, and it hit me how many identical photos of bodies, almost naked bodies, part of bodies, legs, boobs, bums are there—I was completely shocked!"

"When I developed an eating disorder at seventeen, I used images of girls with thigh gaps and thin, ringed fingers in luxe settings—mined from Tumblr, Instagram, Pinterest, and others—to spur my self-starvation. I kept seeing them in my feeds (ironic language there, huh?), wondering when I'd feel as pretty as they appeared to feel."

"The other day at the gym I opened Instagram and said to myself, 'Do you want to look like that or (to the mirror) like that.' That made me spend another thirty minutes on the treadmill."

"I've dabbled in blogging and have tried to grow my own following. I can't help but notice those beautiful girls with large followings and very little to say. I'm willing to bet that if I looked more like them that I would be much more successful in that realm."

"For some people who are already insecure about their looks, social media is pretty much the worst, because it forces you to deal with your looks every single day. It's hard to take a 'break' from thinking about the way you look, because every time you log into Instagram or Facebook you see how fun and gorgeous (at least to you) everyone else looks, and you feel like you can't and won't ever measure up."

BEYOND
BEAUTIFUL
TOOLBOX

The unfollow list

Articles about the impact of social media on our self-esteem often refer to the fact that, compared to other media outlets, we're using social media at a much higher rate (millennials check their phone 150 times a day, apparently), which means that all those harmful, idealized messages reach us at a higher rate, too. But what those articles tend to forget is that social media also has one important advantage over all other media outlets: it is entirely your choice whose messages you allow into your world and whose you leave out.

"Social media is a self-curated bubble. You create your own bubble and then you live in it."

You have a very powerful tool at your disposal to create your very own body image—friendly social media experience: the unfollow button.

Use it liberally on:

- Accounts that make you feel bad about your body or your life

- Attractive people that you follow for no reason other than wanting to stare at them

- People you follow to motivate yourself to change something about the way you look

- Fitness accounts that promote exercise as a means to manage how your body looks rather than how it feels

- Food accounts that you follow as motivation to restrict or monitor your eating

- Beauty accounts that focus on using makeup and other beauty products to improve your appearance, rather than the creativity and self-care aspect of it

- Fashion accounts that value outfits looking on-trend, appropriate, or (the worst) flattering instead of promoting fashion as a way to self-express and have fun

- Accounts that rate, compare, or scrutinize women

- Accounts that otherwise promote the message that beauty equals worth

- Companies that aren't showing any attempts to represent women of different shapes, ages, and ethnicities in their ads

CHAPTER 9

FOOD & FITNESS

Like many women, I've always thought of my body as a work-in-progress. I was always on some sort of plan: to lose weight, to maintain my weight, to tone up (whatever that means), to grow some body part, shrink another. Periods where I'd eat without any guidelines were "breaks" until I'd eventually get "back on track." My New Year's resolutions always included an appearance-related goal.

And up until very recently, I never thought there was a problem with that. And why would I? From makeover TV shows to detoxes, fitness challenges, and endless before-and-afters—all of these things suggest that our bodies are projects with a baseline, a target, and trackable key performance indicators that we can (and should) optimize, manage, and control through food and exercise.

How healthy eating became a status symbol

For decades, our food choices happily resided in the private realm. Sure, there were food trends, and people might try to impress their neighbors with a fancy Sunday brunch once in a while, but for the most part, what you ate was your own business.

Now, things are a little different: what you eat says something about you as a person. The social media churn of leafy greens and sprouted grains artfully arranged on mini plates, actresses talking about their diets, and models showing us how to make smoothies in a five-hundred-dollar blender has firmly established "healthy eating" as yet another box to tick to qualify as a respectable woman.

On top of that comes the fact that, thanks to the internet, we have never been more flooded with information about the dangers of carbs, fats, sugars, gluten, dairy, soy, night-shade plants, and more. So, not only does the food we eat shape our identity, but it could also send us straight into an early grave. Talk about high stakes.

And high stakes lead to high pressure to eat the right way—the good way—all the time. "One night I ate an entire box of sugary cereal and when my friend asked what I'd had for dinner I lied and said I had sushi because I was so embarrassed. I feel like I shouldn't be eating like this at my age," said one woman in my survey. "I eat reasonably healthy, but Instagram makes me feel like a total slob," said another.

Neither of these women is worried about her diet for health reasons—but for identity reasons. They already know that not eating healthfully 100 percent of the time is not going to kill them, but they still feel shame and guilt for not being "the type of woman" who eats nothing but organic produce, tempeh, and superfoods—because in social media culture, healthy (Instagrammable) eating has turned into a status symbol.

And that's bad, because it chucks yet another thing onto the already sky-high mountain of stuff women have to get under control in order to feel like they are doing okay.

Yes, some types of foods are healthier than others, and I am not suggesting you shouldn't eat your veggies or swap your green juice for caramel milkshakes every day. What I am saying is that we as a culture need to stop attaching a moral value to food.

Because just like there is nothing shameful or embarrassing about not always going for the healthiest option in other areas of life (like not getting eight hours of sleep, forgetting to floss, or drinking margaritas on the weekend), there is nothing shameful or embarrassing about eating a box of cereal for dinner once in a while.

A serial dieter's guide to making peace with food

I'm fascinated by people for whom food is a total nonissue, who eat what they want, when they want, without feeling guilty, second-guessing their choices, or thinking about calories or macro- or micronutrients. I'm pretty sure that I used to be one of them, but at some point food stopped being one of the fun, easy things in life and turned into one more thing to master, to get right.

The majority of women that I talked to for this book said they, too, would classify their relationship with food as "complicated." "When I brush my teeth at night I will give myself a grade for how good I've been food-wise that day," said one woman in her thirties. "I started doing it as a teenager and now it just happens automatically—I'm not even trying to lose weight." Many women in my survey were restricting or monitoring their food choices in some way or another. Some were following a specific eating plan, from paleo to alternate-day fasting, or had set themselves food rules, like "only salads for lunch" or "no carbs after 5 pm." Others were counting their calories, carbs, or sugars, had designated certain foods as "cheat food" or completely off-limits, would skip meals when they felt they'd overeaten, or regularly step on the scale to keep their weight "in check."

Now, while some of those things may be sound advice (in some situations) from a physical health standpoint, when it comes to our mental health, they are problematic for one major reason: dieting of any kind messes up your natural, healthy relationship with food.

Plenty of research has backed this up, but perhaps the most famous study that showed this effect is the Minnesota semistarvation experiment from 1944, where thirty-six of the most physically and mentally stable young men were put on a diet of 1,600 calories for six months. Although the researchers were primarily interested in the physical effects of such a low-calorie diet (they were trying to find efficient rations in case of famine), the mental effects turned out to be even more fascinating. "[They] were obsessed with food. They talked about it. They'd spend an inordinate amount of time planning out what they would eat and how they would distribute their calories throughout the day," writes Josie Spinardi in her book, *How to Have Your Cake and Your Skinny Jeans Too!* "They started collecting cookbooks. We're talking young college men—guys with no previous unusual or particular interest in food—who are now spending every free moment ogling *Good Housekeeping* recipes."

You've probably experienced the mind-altering effects of dieting firsthand: once you start imposing rules on yourself, anything edible suddenly looks a lot more delicious than it used to. You think about food all the time and count down the hours until you're allowed to eat again. And once you've fallen off the wagon or decide to get off the diet, all hell breaks loose. Your coworker offers you a slice of birthday cake? You are finishing that thing despite still being stuffed from lunch. Your boyfriend suggests something healthy for dinner? Hell no, pizza is followed by two desserts. You've already broken the diet, so what does it matter? Better make the most of it while you can.

The next morning you're mad at yourself—at your body for producing all these unhelpful cravings and at your brain for having no discipline. But really, it's neither your body nor your brain's fault. All those cravings, that fixation on food and lack of willpower, are simply natural physiological responses to restriction—which, if you're a woman, you likely have a lot of experience with.

The end of the food war:
Intuitive eating

If you're stressed out from food rules dictating your life or just wish you could go back to simpler times, when food was just delicious and not something that could make or break how you feel about yourself, try intuitive eating.

Intuitive eating is a method that was developed by Evelyn Tribole and Elyse Resch in the 1990s to help people like you and me revert back to a natural, nonstressful relationship with food, by relearning how to trust our body's built-in control system: our hunger.

Here's how it works: You eat exactly what you want to eat when you are hungry. You don't eat when you are not hungry. That's it. Sounds simple? Yep. This is how kids, animals, and adult humans who somehow managed to remain unaffected by our diet culture eat. But for someone like me, who's got years of dieting under her belt, eating like this takes guts.

"Eating in abandon and trusting that the body will actually begin to pipe up is one of the scariest things an ex-dieter can do, but it is also one of the most healing. We believe the body is always trying to lead us astray, and the most healing thing I've ever learned, is that all the body wants to do is communicate with you and help you thrive," says Caroline Dooner, fellow ex—serial dieter and author of *The F*ck It Diet*. Plenty of studies have backed this up and shown that even people with a long history of dieting or binge eating can learn to eat intuitively, which leads to a whole bunch of good stuff: more body satisfaction, less anxiety around food, no more bingeing, and no more thinking about food all the time.

What is your relationship with food?

"I grew up in Australia but hated going to the beach because I didn't want anyone to see my body. I have been on weight-loss programs on and off since I was twelve. It's always something that's in the back of my mind—this idea that if I lost weight and had a perfect body then my life would be easier and better."

"Diets are a slippery slope for me. I have slipped into very unhealthy eating tendencies, from bingeing to the point of being ill, to starving myself for a few days, all starting as young as eight years old."

"I am careful with what I eat—some would say certainly fanatical. I don't eat grain, dairy, corn, potatoes, pork, fast food, chocolate, nuts, or beans, EVER. That's the only way I can keep my weight at the same it was when I was a teen."

"For most of my life, I prided myself on being the 'skinny girl who could eat whatever she wanted.' But deep down inside, I was obsessed with gaining weight and terrified of being too skinny. I wanted curves and to feel womanly."

"I have been on every diet ever invented and none of them worked. I call everything related to food 'the food war.' Tracking does make you aware of what you are eating but makes you think about food constantly."

"I often fall into cycles where I hype myself up to eat as little as possible and skip every meal I can without anyone noticing."

"I'm always on a program of some sort. I've struggled with binge eating, so I'm often on the hamster wheel of the bingeing/restricting cycle."

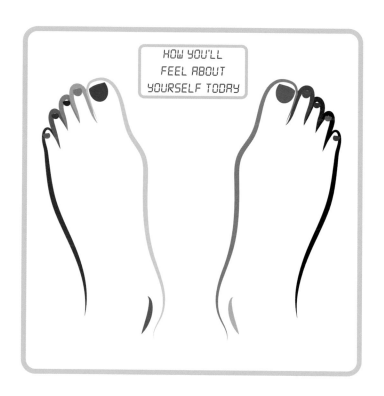

For me, intuitive eating has been a game changer. Before, I could never understand why someone would just choose to leave half of their chocolate desert just sitting there. Like, you have the option to eat that, you are not on a diet, so why in the world would you not finish it? Now, after a while on the intuitive-eating train and simply eating what I want without setting myself any rules, I recently even forgot all about a delicious piece of carrot cake that I'd had in a doggy bag until I rediscovered it in my purse a week later. In the past, that would have *never* happened.

INTUITIVE EATING 101

- Eat when you are hungry.

- Eat whatever you most feel like eating.

- Keep a wide variety of foods available so you'll have exactly what you feel like eating when you need it.

- Limit planning meals far in advance.

- Stop eating when you feel full.*

- Don't eat when you're not hungry, even if it's mealtime.*

At the beginning, it's crucial that you get out of the restriction mind-set, so don't worry about these last two points too much.

PSA: It's time to ditch your scale for good

For years I was a slave to my bathroom scale: I would step on it every morning, sometimes several times a day, then hold my breath and wait for the little numbers to pop up, to tell me if my day was going to be a good one or not. A lower number than I expected would make me feel ecstatic. A higher number could ruin my whole day.

A majority of the women in my research said that for them, too, stepping on the scale is a terrifying act of self-flagellation. And yet, they keep doing it because it gives them a sense of control. The mirror lies and photos are too inconsistent, but a scale gives them the objectivity—a clear judgment about the way their body looks—that they so crave.

The problem is, of course, that a scale doesn't actually have anything meaningful to say about the way your body looks. Your weight fluctuates constantly based on so many factors, from how much water you have been drinking to your hormones, your cycle, how much food is in your stomach, what position the scale is standing in on the floor. When you are working out, that list gets even longer: you may be gaining muscle, you may be holding on to water, you may be dehydrated, and so on. To base your whole assessment of your body on such an unreliable measurement is crazy.

And guess what: you don't need to know how much you weigh. Unless you are an athlete who needs to stay in a weight class, your body's exact gravitational force down to the pound has zero relevance.

"But if I don't weigh myself, then I'm just going to balloon!" Well, no. Just because you're no longer monitoring your scale weight does not mean you're signing a blank check for your body to defy the laws of physics and do what it wants. You are still going to see yourself in the mirror every day, and you'll notice any meaningful weight changes by the way your clothes fit. But you'll no longer get worked up over the meaningless weight changes that used to take up so much of your energy.

The problem with exercising to "look better naked"

We're in the middle of a fitness craze and more people than ever are hitting the gym, getting sweaty on the regular, and working toward #fitnessgoals. And on the surface, it may seem like our collective approach to fitness has shifted to a more body image—friendly level. We have moved on from one-pound dumbbells and counting calories. We no longer want to be skinny; we want to be fit, strong, and healthy!

But underneath our quest for "wellness," it's easy to still spot our appearance focus. Studies have shown that the language used on "fitspiration" social media accounts is often barely distinguishable from that used on pro-anorexia websites. It's about control, pushing yourself, stigmatizing your "before" body, praising yourself and others for restraint, and loading a whole bunch of meaning onto the way your body looks. In the end, #fitnessgoals is just a euphemism for #appearancegoals.

And ironically, exercising to feel better about the way you look can quite easily do the opposite. Here's why.

The carrot and the stick

When your number one reason for working out is to change the way your body looks, you'll approach the whole thing in a very different way than you would if you were training for the challenge, for a competition, or simply for fun. You may choose to take up running because that is supposed to burn lots of calories, sign up for barre class because you want "long, lean muscles," or shell out for some fitness guru's "abs and booty program."

Now, if you love running, barre, and whatever "abs and booty programs" entail, all of that is great, but if you don't, then you'll need to constantly motivate yourself to stick to your program. And guess what your motivation will be? Yep, all of your physical shortcomings and how much you want to "fix" them. When you hit a wall in your workout, you'll push yourself to keep going by thinking about how much you hate your jiggly thighs. When it's rainy outside, you'll convince yourself to put on your running shoes by fantasizing about how great you'll feel once your stomach is flat and your upper arms less flabby.

That's just the way we've all learned to motivate ourselves: by focusing on our goals, on how much we want the carrot and hate the stick, and by hyping ourselves up a little. And sure, all that hype may well make you stick to your routine, but it also turns every workout into a mental reinforcement of your insecurities, and your status quo body into the enemy.

The magnifying glass

When you think of exercise as part of your beauty routine, your measure of progress will be physical change. But of course, physical changes don't happen overnight, so you'll need to keep close tabs on the way your body looks to spot them. You need to keep pinching your arm fat to see if those spinning classes are making a difference. You need to pay close attention to your glutes to make sure they are responding to your lifting routine. You need to keep flexing your abs to check if you're any closer to a two-pack than you were last week.

That type of hyperfocus on your body acts like a magnifying glass. You'll eventually know every inch of your body so well that you lose sight of it. Your "flaws" appear more prominent and tiny changes seem major. Every move in the right direction gives you a dopamine hit that leaves you craving more. You may find yourself staring at the mirror for minutes at a time trying to spot "progress," use every shop window as an opportunity to inspect your new form, or take pictures of yourself to get a better sense of what you look like.

And even if you eventually reach your goal, you still won't be satisfied—because that magnifying glass is still there, showing you plenty more to nitpick. Instead of overcoming your insecurities, you've been feeding them all along.

"I think in today's society there is a lack of movement for movement's sake—as an adult, all physical activity is 'exercise'—which means that we cannot appreciate our body for the miracle it is, something that allows us to reach and run and twist and bend."

"When I took up heavy resistance training, the way I saw myself changed completely. It simply feels empowering to be able to physically overcome difficult tasks."

REFLECTION QUESTIONS

What is your motivation to work out?

What makes a "good" workout for you? How do you measure progress?

If exercise had no effect on the way you look whatsoever, would you still work out the way you do right now? If, not what would you change?

CHAPTER 10

STYLE

Clothes and body image are inextricably linked. It's hard to have fun with fashion or even just feel good about your day-to-day outfits when full-length mirrors send you into a low-grade panic. To make matters worse, in the media, fashion is still presented in much the same way as women's bodies: something that you need to get right with clear-cut rules. It's no wonder clothing stores can feel like such a minefield.

In this chapter we'll talk about how to stop your body image from preventing you from dressing in a way that you love. But, just for the record, you can wear plastic bags every day of the week if you want to, if you feel good in them. I am in no way suggesting that to improve your body image you have to spend time or money on your clothes. If your clothes are not a problem for you, then great! This chapter is for the rest of us:

- Who feel like they can't wear the clothes they want because of how their body looks

- Who believe there's no point in wearing nice clothes because they are going to look bad anyway

- Who worry about their outfits looking unflattering, basic, inappropriate, or just not cool enough

The importance of wearing what you like no matter your body image

For the longest time my closet contained two very different sets of clothes: my *thin* clothes and my *fat* clothes. My thin clothes were colorful and had cool patterns and interesting cuts. They were fun to wear, reflected my personality, and made me want to get extra creative with accessories, hairstyles, and makeup. If I could have, I would have worn my thin clothes all the time. The dilemma: I could only fit into them after at least two months of intense dieting and almost-daily gym sessions. For the rest of the time, I had my fat clothes.

My fat clothes were only about one or two sizes larger than my thin clothes, but they looked like they belonged to a different person: bulky sweaters, dark colors, ill-fitting jeans, and T-shirts in various shades of gray. Although I was probably wearing my fat clothes at least two-thirds of the time, they only made up about 10 percent of my closet. That's because I would only ever buy clothes when I was "thin." Buying clothes that I liked when I wasn't happy about my body never even occurred to me; I thought, "I'm going to look bad anyway, so what's the point?"

Many people in my survey told me about following a similar all-or-nothing logic when it comes to clothes, about feeling like there is no point in wearing what they like until they have lost five, fifteen, or fifty pounds, or they've gotten the boob job, or their face has cleared up. For a lot of women, feeling like this isn't even a temporary situation. All they know is they don't like the way they look right now, so nice clothes would be lost on them anyway.

> "I sometimes fantasize about what I'd wear if I had my dream body, and I even put clothes in the cart online. I'm not sure why I do this; I guess I like torturing myself."

The reason so many of us feel this way is because we have fully lapped up the idea that the whole purpose of our clothes is to make us look more attractive. It is a simple extension of the self-objectifying perspective we use to judge our body: we take on what we believe is the perspective of others and evaluate ourselves from their point of view, because that is what we have been taught really counts.

Our clothes are just another area where this idea is making our lives harder than it has to be. Because when we stop thinking of clothes as a tool for managing how *others* see us, they can turn into something that pleases *ourselves*. This is a way to create a space for ourselves wherever we go, to feel comfortable and ready to tackle whatever life throws at us, and to self-express, be creative, and have fun with colors and shapes just like an artist would, if we are into that.

For me, this approach was one of the biggest revelations that I came to while working on this book. Bit by bit, as I stopped dieting, I started buying clothes that I love just as much as my thin clothes, just in a bigger size. Because I finally understood that there are no two versions of me, the thin version and the fat version, that both are equally just me—a person who loves color, patterns, interesting cuts, and who deserves to wear exactly what she wants to wear.

To what extent does your body image prevent you from wearing what you like at the moment?

What would you wear if you had a perfect body image?

Stop dressing for your "body type"

I once sat next to a group of girls on a train, all of them twelve, perhaps thirteen years old. One of them wanted to buy a new pair of jeans, and she talked about what kind she might want to get. "I don't like high-waisted jeans but I have to wear them because I'm a pear shape." she said. "Just make sure you get black or dark blue ones to make your legs look smaller. And wear that with something white on top to balance it out," said one of the other girls. "I wish I was an apple shape. That way I couldn't wear tight tops, but at least I could wear dresses and short shorts. That's good for the summer." They all agreed.

That whole situation seems so absurd to me now, even though I remember when I was their age, I was also already very aware of my body type, my "flaws" and "assets." And that's because for decades now the concept of "dressing for your body shape" has been everywhere—a staple in fashion magazines, on blogs, and on makeover shows that is so commonly accepted, even twelve-year-olds know their "type."

Ironically, it's often presented as confidence-boosting, as something you should do for yourself, to "celebrate" your unique shape, when really the goal is the exact opposite: it blatantly promotes the idea that the first and foremost objective of clothes is to manipulate, hide, or minimize your body.

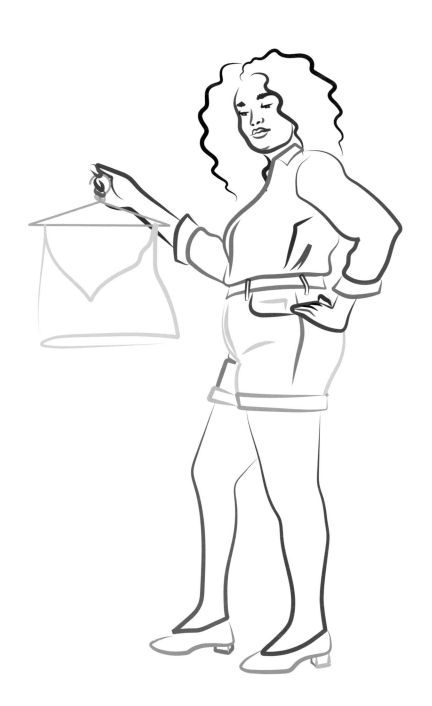

Think about it. Dressing for your shape is all about choosing clothes that "flatter" your body. To "flatter" means nothing but "makes you look thinner, taller, more curvy or less curvy," whichever side your body falls on in comparison to what's currently considered "ideal."

Figuring out your body type is also a terribly in-depth exercise in something that most women already do way too much of: nitpicking. I remember I once had a book that listed twelve different body types, and my friends and I would spend whole afternoons trying to figure out if our waists were "gently sloping" enough for our bodies to be considered a lollipop or a vase, and whether broad shoulders meant we were a goblet or a cornet.

"I hate when shop assistants try to convince me to buy their clothes by telling me how much slimmer I look. Who says I want to look slimmer?"

Then, once you've figured out your type, you are given a set of rules for how to dress. For example, a typical recommendation for the pear shape might go something like this: "Find clothes that enhance your waist because that is your smallest part (smallest = best), and go for A-line cut skirts and dresses that skim over your wide hips and thighs (wide = must be minimized) to make your body seem more proportionate" (as if a pear-shaped body, perhaps the most common female body type, is somehow disproportionate and must be altered to look okay).

The ubiquity of the idea that our clothes should be "appropriate" for our body type reflects the scary extent to which we have all internalized that looking slim and attractive according to today's societal ideals is much more important than wearing clothes you personally like, self-expression, and having fun with fashion.

The girls on the train did not for one second talk about which types of jeans they liked or wanted to wear; they talked about which types of jeans would make their legs seem smaller and which jeans they were "allowed" to wear. And they were all in total agreement about it, none of them questioning whether looking skinny should even be such a concern to them—as if it's just a no-brainer, just something that you do as a female.

Of course you should feel confident in whatever you are wearing. Definitely! But I believe that confidence should stem from the fact that you love your outfit because it reflects your personal style, your personality, or your opinions, or simply because you find it ridiculously comfortable and it serves you well during your day-to-day life, and not because it makes you look two pounds lighter or half an inch taller.

So, if I could send those girls from the train a message, it would be this: Wear clothes that you like! Wear clothes that feel good, that feel like "you." And forget about all the rest of the stuff—body shapes, what supposedly flatters you, all that. If you don't like high-waisted jeans, don't wear them— even if you are a pear shape and have been told your whole life that low-waisted cuts don't work with your hips. If somebody tells you what you're wearing doesn't flatter you, ignore them. It's not your job to look as close as possible to whatever's currently considered ideal.

Wear whatever you like. And let's all just stop using the word "flattering," okay?

Do you try to dress for your body type?

Is there anything you would wear if you had a completely different body type?

What keeps you from wearing that now?

Stop dressing for your age

While we are on the topic of silly fashion rules: please feel free to ignore any and all advice you have ever heard about dressing age-appropriately. Guidelines like "no miniskirts after forty" are among the last sticky leftovers of antiquated gender roles telling women how to behave in order to be a respectable member of society, in the same vein as telling women to make sure to be married by the time they are thirty, or they'll end up as a sad spinster.

Your age should not limit your ability to dress your body the way you want, even if the majority of people your age dress differently.

Stop wearing uncomfortable clothes

As women, we grow up with this idea that discomfort is just the price we have to pay for looking chic, feminine, and put-together. And so we grind our teeth and spend day after day wearing bras that dig into our skin, jeans that almost cut off our circulation, and skirts that have us wobbling from point A to point B. For special occasions we're willing to trade in even more physical well-being and mobility in exchange for a few extra chicness points: four-inch-heels, extra-tight dresses, shapewear, and so on.

All of that discomfort costs energy and keeps us from being able to fully enjoy the moment. I learned this the hard way when I got invited to an art exhibition and decided to splurge on some new heels because I wanted to look extra chic that day. I knew those heels were probably not going to be comfy, but I was sure I would be fine—this was a fancy event, after all, and the majority of women were going to be in heels. Unfortunately, after about ten minutes, it became apparent that I would not be "fine." When the artist talked us through her pieces I could barely pay attention because I was so focused on trying to shift my weight in an effort to relieve the burning pain in the balls of my feet at least a tiny bit. I had been so excited about that exhibition, but, in the end, I left early and walked barefoot to the closest taxi stand.

After that experience I made the conscious decision to no longer put up with uncomfortable clothes—not for everyday life and not even for special occasions. I got rid of all of my too-tight clothes, any shoes that would give me blisters, and every single pokey bra that would leave my back covered in red marks by the end of the night. That decision was a result of me being fed up at the time, but in retrospect I can see that it also did wonders for my body image.

Each time we wear uncomfortable clothes for aesthetic reasons or even just to conform to a social norm (such as wearing heels for evening events), we reinforce our own belief that how we are perceived by others is more important that our own well-being. When we stop wearing uncomfortable clothes, we accomplish the opposite: we tell our subconscious that our ability to fully experience, enjoy, and interact with the world is what's key. If we can wear cute clothes while doing that, fine. But our well-being comes first.

Life is too short for uncomfortable clothes.

REFLECTION QUESTIONS ───────────────

Do you regularly wear items that you find uncomfortable?

How does wearing uncomfortable clothes affect your mood?

The body confidence closet makeover

I'm a fan of extreme makeovers as long as they involve changing clothes instead of body parts. All you need is about two-hours and a couple of bags to house the garments you're not keeping until have time to donate, sell, or repurpose them. Throw fashion rules, body type guidelines, and other "shoulds" and "shouldn'ts" out the window, then go through your entire closet piece-by-piece.

Thanks, but no!

- Clothes that don't fit you

- Clothes that you're keeping as motivation to hit the gym

- Clothes you wear to hide your "flaws"

- Clothes that you only bought because they supposedly "flatter" your body type

- Clothes that you want to take off as soon as you get home

- Clothes you can barely move in

- Clothes you have to readjust every five minutes

Oh yes, please!

- Clothes that put you in a happy mood

- Clothes that express your personality, opinions, or interests

- Cuts that fit the individual contours of your body without tugging or digging in

- Colors you've always loved

- Fabrics that feel amazing on your skin

- Clothes you can run, jump, and dance in

- Clothes that make you forget you're even wearing anything

CHAPTER 11

BEAUTY ROUTINES

I've been "into beauty" ever since I first lay hands on *Bobbi Brown's Teenage Beauty* at age fourteen. Since then, like so many women, I've spent a considerable amount of time, energy, and money on my beauty routine.

Just for a regular weekday, I spend more time getting ready than my boyfriend does in a full week. My bathroom is full of pretty lotions and potions. I have no idea what my underarm hair looks like in its full glory because from the moment it first started sprouting, I've been attacking every last bit with a razor, and I don't think I've left the house without at least some makeup on my face for at least ten years. A big chunk of my money goes toward beauty products, tools, and treatments, and a big chunk of my free time each week is carved out for "maintenance," including at-home facials, doing my nails, hair removal, lashes, eyebrows, all that jazz.

The thing is, in our culture, being preoccupied with beauty like I was is not only *not* frowned upon but often encouraged and expected. Dedication when it comes to sticking to your routine is considered a high virtue, and we nod in agreement when magazine editors and beauty gurus instruct us to "Never *ever* go to bed with makeup on!"

But could it be that instead of making us feel better about ourselves, our approach to beauty is making us feel worse?

Is your beauty routine boycotting your body image?

As we have discussed, no action in and of itself is bad for your body image—it's the thought process behind it that counts. The same goes for all things beauty. A minimal routine is neither an indicator of a perfect body image, nor is it somehow superior to wearing a full face of makeup on a daily basis.

You can use beauty products in all sorts of positive ways: If you love being creative, makeup and hair-styling can be amazing outlets. Skin and body care can be a way to relax, have a little "me time," and connect with your body, all of which are very helpful for body image.

What's not great for your body image is when you are using beauty products as a coping mechanism, because they give you a sense of control and make you feel better about your insecurities. When your routine is growing ever more complex as you try to chase society's demands; when you are pushing yourself to complete your full routine, even when you'd much rather be doing something else; when you are using your beauty routine as a crutch instead of dealing with your body-image issues head-on.

A beauty routine like that not only validates your insecurities, but it also feeds them in the long run by changing how you look at your body. Just like having an intense focus on diet and exercise, being super into beauty makes you look at your body in a different, hyperfocused way that acts like a magnifying glass over your features. Once you pay attention to small details on your face, such as fine lines, it's only a small step until you notice other things on the same level of focus, like uneven eyebrows or large pores. You start seeing your body as something you have the power to optimize, rather than something that is just there. You're opening the floodgates to envisioning all the things that *could* be. You turn into an interior designer who wants to redecorate every room she walks into. Or a copywriter who can't read a laundromat flyer without thinking of all the ways that sales pitch could have been stronger. Once you've dipped your toe into the wondrous power of beauty, it's only a matter of time until you find more and more about yourself that could be optimized.

Plus, if you don't enjoy doing any of those things, they are also just a major waste of life. Imagine if instead of having to spend an hour in the bathroom every morning, you could choose to just spend ten minutes and use the extra time to work on a personal project, play with your dog, or just chill on the couch and read a book. Sounds good, right?

Of course, it's totally possible, and very likely, that you are using beauty products for both positive and negative reasons right now. In that case, we'll work on separating the wheat from the chaff in the next steps. For now, just analyze your status quo.

Do you enjoy your beauty routine in the moment? Are there parts you look forward to?

Do you sometimes feel like your beauty routine is taking up too much of your time?

Do you worry about spending too much money on beauty products or treatments?

Has your beauty routine expanded over time?

Do you often notice more things to fix about your skin, hair, or face?

Have your standards inflated? (Did you have a goal and when you reached it, were you still not happy?)

Does your beauty routine sometimes feel like a chore? Which steps? Do you still make yourself do them when you don't want to?

Fun and flexible: What a confident approach to beauty looks like

So what does a healthy beauty routine look like from a body-image perspective? Compared to a typical chaser's packed and insecurity-driven routine, it is defined by two things.

Pleasure-driven, not fear-driven

Instead of using beauty products from a place of fear—to cover up "flaws" or fix what you feel self-conscious about—you do things because they are fun or feel good in the moment. Instead of letting your insecurities run the show and trying to change your appearance to please *others*, you use your beauty routine as a way to please *yourself*.

How does your body image affect your beauty routine?

"I always put on makeup. I don't have to think about how I would feel if I didn't do it because that would NEVER happen. Never ever!"

"I usually go out completely natural, and I love it. It is so freeing to just be like, 'Here I am, world, take it or leave it.'"

"I'm fanatical about sunscreen! If I forget to put on sunscreen, everything has to stop until I go back and put it on. Taking care of my skin is at the top of my priorities—sunscreen is a must!"

"I have blonde eyelashes and brows, so I always wear mascara and do my eyebrows. If I don't, people usually ask me if I'm sick or tired."

"It feels freeing to not do any beauty stuff—but then that often makes me feel invisible, like I'm self-shaming. Not even respecting myself to do the things I want to do—cute makeup, nails, expressive outfit."

"In some ways I take pride in not caring about my appearance. I teach, and it matters to me that my young students see that I am comfortable without makeup and fashion."

"I once had to give a presentation at work on a day I wasn't wearing makeup. I felt a bit uncomfortable in the beginning, but then forgot about it. The audience was not there to look at me, but to listen to what I was saying."

FEAR-DRIVEN

- Spending a ton of cash on expensive skin care products because you are terrified of wrinkles and other signs of aging

- Manicuring your nails every three days because you don't want anyone judging you for looking "unkempt"

- Wearing a full face of makeup every day because you feel plain and unattractive without it

PLEASURE-DRIVEN

- Treating yourself to a facial because it relaxes you

- Wearing nail polish because you like the color

- Spending a long time on your makeup because you love the creative aspect of it

Of course, there are some things that just aren't fun, but you may still choose to do, like shaving your legs. In these cases, it is important to consider the next aspect of healthy beauty routines.

Flexible, not nonnegotiable

Everything in a healthy beauty routine is optional, not a must. One day you may feel like taking the time to go all out with your makeup, other days you may skip it. A flexible beauty routine allows for your different moods, schedules, and so on. You know that even if you don't do something, you are still the same person and still worth the same.

NONNEGOTIABLE

- Shaving your legs every day because you can't bear the thought of tiny stubble

- Not leaving the house without having done your brows, foundation, and concealer

- Sticking to your waxing schedule religiously because you're worried your partner could get freaked out by a bit of extra hair "down there"

FLEXIBLE

- Shaving your legs when you have time in the morning

- Skipping your regular makeup routine from time to time to sleep in an extra fifteen minutes

- Canceling your waxing appointment when you'd rather meet a friend for lunch

REFLECTION QUESTIONS ———————————

Which steps in your beauty routine do you enjoy? Are there any things you would enjoy but are not yet doing?

Are there any aspects of your beauty routine that are nonnegotiable? What would happen if you skipped them?

The Beyond Beautiful reset challenge

A good way to transition from a strict nonnegotiable beauty routine to a more flexible, pleasure-driven routine is with a little beauty reset.

The goal of this exercise is to help you reset what you currently consider your "normal" self. If you only ever see your bare skin and lashes at the end of the day, then of course you'll start to associate your bare face with feeling tired and blah, and end up believing that you need to put your "face" on before you can accomplish anything.

The other point of this exercise is to give yourself the chance to notice that nothing bad actually happens when you stop your grooming routine. People treat you the same way they did before, your cats still love you, your friends still talk to you—it's all good.

For seven days, keep your beauty routine to an absolute minimum: do things that get you clean and keep you physically comfortable. You can wash and moisturize your face, wash and moisturize your body, wash and condition your hair, brush your teeth and hair, and use deodorant. But except for that, *nada*.

Daily check-in

Keep a mini diary throughout the week, answering these questions:

- On a scale of 1 to 10, how confident did you feel about your minimally groomed self today?

- Did you feel self-conscious at any point during the day? Why?

- Were there any parts of your day that went better than expected?

Post-reset reflection

After the seven days are over, reflect on your experience using these questions:

- Was the week easier or harder than you had expected? Why?

- What were the biggest challenges you ran into?

- Did you notice any practical benefits to having a stripped-down routine?

- How did the reset affect your confidence levels throughout the week?

- What type of situations were you in when you felt self-conscious during the week? Who were you with?

- When you felt self-conscious, what exactly was your thought process? Did you worry that others would think of you in a different way, that they'd make comments?

- Were there any steps in your routine that you thought you'd feel super self-conscious without, but were actually fine with leaving out?

- Were there any aspects of your routine that you missed doing (not for the result, just for the process)?

Rebuilding your routine

After your beauty reset, you will have hopefully learned some new things about yourself, experienced the freedom of not having to do stuff you don't like, and also noticed which aspects of your routine you actually missed, because you simply enjoy the process. Based on that information, you can now put together your very own pleasure-driven and flexible beauty routine.

Now, instead of listing every single step (remember: your beauty routine is not a to-do list; everything is optional), ask yourself two questions:

1. WHAT DO I WANT TO DO LESS OFTEN?

What stuff do you hate doing? What takes too long, what's painful, or what do you do only to please others or conform to societal standards? Write down everything you want to spend less time doing in the future or scrap from your routine entirely.

2. WHAT DO I WANT TO DO MORE OFTEN?

Which parts of your routine do you enjoy? What did you miss during your one-week reset? And what would you like to try for fun?

"If you retain nothing else, always remember the most important rule of beauty, which is: who cares?"

Tina Fey, *Bossypants*

CHAPTER 12

COSMETIC SURGERY

Only a decade ago, cosmetic surgery was a hush-hush topic. Now, magazines review the newest procedures the same way they review designer collections, and people openly talk about trying out lip fillers for fun and how their boob job was the best thing they ever did for themselves. Celebrities used to come under fire for getting plastic surgery; nowadays, no one bats an eye when teenage celebrities show up with a whole new face and become social media stars with beauty empires.

When it comes to women's body image, cosmetic surgery is a tricky subject—especially because it needs to be looked at from two separate perspectives: that of the individual and that of society as a whole. So let's investigate!

The normalization of "getting work done": Harmful, helpful, or no big deal?

In my survey, no other question sparked more divergent answers than whether the normalization of cosmetic procedures (whether we're talking the invasive kind or stuff like fillers and Botox) is helping or hurting women's body image. Many women had a crystal-clear opinion: "I will never cut or inject anything in or on my body unless it is medically necessary. I can actually get enraged at doctors profiting from women's insecurities."

Others looked at the whole idea from a more pragmatic perspective: "If something constantly bothers you, and it cannot realistically be tackled otherwise, why not get it surgically fixed? Many people spend tons on ineffective magic creams to start with. It's more cost-effective in the long term to just get plastic surgery and be done with it."

And sure, there is no denying that for some people, cosmetic surgery can end years of suffering. One woman wrote to me: "I had a huge overbite (eleven millimeters) and when I finally got surgery at eighteen, it was like I was a new person overnight."

But for society as a whole, the normalization of cosmetic surgery is bad news. Of course, we want to live in a world where women can do what they want with their bodies without being judged. But if more and more women sport perfectly sculpted noses, ultra-smooth foreheads in their fifties, or perky boobs after pregnancy, it undoubtedly creates a new baseline and pushes our already unrealistic beauty ideals even further through the roof.

What's worse is that the vast majority of those who shape our society's beauty standards—A-listers, models, and other people in the public eye—do not disclose the fact that they've had cosmetic surgery. I have a friend who has a real obsession with people's noses because of her insecurities with her own. She is convinced that 95 percent of Hollywood actresses—including those who you'd never expect it from—have had a nose job. Whether her estimate is correct or not, I'm going to go out on a limb here and say that it's at least likely that way more people in the public eye have had work done than most of us realize. And even though many celebrities these days have no problem talking about the hours of pre—award show prep, lasers, shapewear, hard-core workouts, even that onetime Botox injection they tried but didn't like, the real whammy—invasive plastic surgery—is still a big black hole.

How do you feel about cosmetic surgery?

"My mother has had a lot of plastic surgery and watching her go through it has been traumatic. It does not help body image; it just sets new unreachable standards."

"I think it's beneficial that people who need or desire cosmetic surgery can now get it without quite so much judgment. It's their house and they should decorate it as they please."

"My breasts have a two-cup size difference, and it would have really helped my thirteen-year-old self if someone had pulled me aside and said, 'If this size difference bothers you so much, there are ways to fix it.'"

"I've had five surgeries in my life—all were to save my life. I feel horrible that so many women would go under general anesthesia to 'improve' themselves."

"My lazy eyelid used to be a huge insecurity for me, but I always thought I was being really vain for being bothered by it so much. When an eye doctor finally told me, 'Wow, this is bad and it can be fixed!' I felt a huge sense of relief because someone finally acknowledged that it's okay for me to be bothered by it, and I'm not just a super vain person."

"As much as I agree that it's your body and you can do what you want, we also don't make choices in a vacuum, and cosmetic surgery becoming a new standard for beauty seems like a self-perpetuating, highly profitable system. So while I don't judge any one woman for getting cosmetic surgery, I'm very critical of the overall system and the subtle ways that we push women toward getting cosmetic surgery and really downplay the risks."

We can get mad at magazine airbrushing all we want, but as long as the people who shape our idea of beauty systematically model a standard that cannot be achieved without major surgery, tens of thousands of dollars, and the willingness (and time) to endure pain, discomfort, and immobility, our collective body image will remain in big trouble.

That's not to say that if everyone suddenly decided to reveal their past nip and tuck list we'd be in a much better position. Yes, it might make us feel a little better about our God-given bodies, but it would still send the message to girls and women everywhere that beauty is a prerequisite to success, and that it warrants all the time, energy, money, and physical discomfort you can afford.

Articles in magazines about the newest high-tech "totally pain-free" procedures and casual "My plastic surgery experience"—type content are problematic for the same reason. By normalizing cosmetic procedures and thereby normalizing the fact that so many people go to great lengths to look better, we raise the value of physical beauty to an even higher level than it already has in our society.

So while we should not judge any individual for choosing to get work done (and that includes Hollywood actresses), we *definitely* should judge and be very critical of a system that makes going under the knife (or needle) seem like your best option in the first place.

Real talk: Would cosmetic surgery improve your confidence?

We all want to be socially responsible and not make life harder for our future daughters, friends, and coworkers, but at the end of the day, the key factor that makes people decide for or against surgery is what they believe it's going to do to for their own life—whether they believe it's going to make them more confident and happier.

Now, there is no point in denying that, for example, getting lipo probably *would* improve your confidence—if the fat on your stomach is the sole reason for your confidence issues (and if all goes well). According to most studies, the majority of cosmetic procedures do produce satisfaction with the body part that was treated. But that *still* doesn't mean cosmetic surgery is a magic bullet when it comes to body image. Because often, that body part you want to get fixed is *not* the cause of your less-than-ideal confidence levels. Your dissatisfaction with it is just a symptom of a much larger issue: a generally low body image.

Getting work done when your overall body image is low is a bad idea for two reasons.

"That's not what I ordered"

Studies have shown that people who have a low body image are less likely to be satisfied with the result of both invasive and noninvasive cosmetic procedures (like Botox and fillers), which is not surprising considering that it's not the body part that's the problem, but rather their per-ception and evaluation of it. For that reason, most good cosmetic surgeons will quiz potential patients about their overall body satisfaction before agreeing to perform a procedure.

It's a slippery slope

Unfortunately, even if you are satisfied with the results of your procedure, you're not out of the woods yet. Because when your body image is less-than-ideal, being happy with your new "look" could very well send you down the much-discussed slippery slope of even more procedures. Let's say you decide to get a nose job. You get it done, and you love the result. You can't stop looking at yourself in the mirror, you take mountains of selfies to admire your nose, and you have tons more confidence around people. You want to go out more, you feel more assertive at work, and you suddenly love it when people take pictures. You are so glad you went through with it. But then, after a while, that elated feeling goes down as you get used to your new nose, and you start feeling self-conscious again. Because your original problem, your low body image, is still there.

"I went for some laser hair removal and fat freezing and came back with a list of other flaws I should address!"

Soon enough you'll attribute those feelings of self-consciousness to another aspect of your appearance, perhaps your thighs this time. Yeah, you never liked those. And so the whole process starts again, except this time, your decision that you want it "fixed" will come easier than before. Your experience the first time around, all of that extra confidence, happiness, and the positive responses from others (which may well have just been reactions to your new happy vibe, instead of your new physical attributes), has only strengthened your belief that beauty equals happiness. Plus, having gone through the process once before, you will have also broken down the natural barrier that people have toward being cut into or injected with something for the sake of beauty. You already went through it once, it was fine, so what's the harm?

You may think, "I don't have to worry about that; I could never afford having multiple things done." But whether you actually go through with a second, third, or fourth surgery is not the point. The point is that having cosmetic surgery once and liking the result could well lead you down a slippery slope of permanent dissatisfaction, always seeing your appearance as a work-in-progress. You may look better but you'll *feel* worse in the long run.

Red flags

Hopefully, after working through this book, you already have a pretty good idea whether your lack of confidence really just stems from one body part or whether your body image as a whole could use some brushing up. But just in case, here are the biggest red flags that point to your general body image needing work more urgently than any of your body parts:

- You barely like anything about your appearance

- You have a whole laundry list of cosmetic procedures you want to get in the future

- You use a lot of coping strategies (running, hiding or chasing)

- You feel like a lesser person because of the way you look

If you really want to get surgery, and your body image is good except for this one thing that's been bothering you for years, and you are prepared to do your due diligence and see multiple doctors until you find someone you click with, then go ahead.

But if you even have an inkling that your desire to "get work done" is a symptom of your generally bad body image, hold off and work on your internal self first. The same goes if you are generally at a crossroads in your life. Once you are in a better place, you may well find that you no longer want to get surgery, because your body dissatisfaction was just a symptom of a larger dip in your life story.

Conclusion:
Weltschmerz and
the squiggly trajectory
of change

There's this great German word, *weltschmerz* (which literally means "world pain"), that perfectly describes how I felt when I first started working on this book and really began to understand the devastating impact our society's looks obsession has on the daily lives of so many women and men around the world.

But eventually, my *weltschmerz* turned into cautious optimism. The first stage of any meaningful cultural shift is always awareness. It's being clear about the fact that things are bad right now and need to change. We've definitely accomplished that. Now we're in the middle of the next hurdle—negotiating the terms of our new and, hopefully, a much-improved approach to beauty—which is also going to take a bit of back and forth. Progress is rarely linear—that goes for societal movements as much as it does for our own personal goals. Just like we as a society will likely keep trying on different perspectives for size, making some wins here and there (like the #MeToo movement), but also taking steps back (like thigh gaps becoming a thing), your personal journey toward a healthy body image will likely be squiggly, too.

As you work through this book, you'll hopefully make steady progress and some huge leaps forward, but you can also expect multiple tiny to substantial setbacks that will have you thinking, "Wow, I thought I'd moved beyond that." The best thing you can do in those situations is to be open and honest—because showing your struggle and letting others in immediately takes the heat off the one thing that underlies all body worries: shame.

And no matter where you are in your body-image journey, don't be afraid to share what you have learned with others. Tell your friends, your mom, your coworkers, your social media followers why it's so important that we as women recalibrate our self-worth barometer, what's problematic about ad slogans encouraging us to look better naked, and how we can thank crafty advertisers for the majority of our unrealistic beauty standards.

Sharing knowledge and ideas not only helps others cut corners on their own squiggly trajectory to body confidence, but it also reminds *you* of all of these things. It reminds you that—just like your friend, your mother, your coworker—you too are beyond beautiful.

Want to see how others are using the tools and advice in this book, or share your own story, thoughts, and experiences? Head over to @beyondbeautifulbook on Instagram! See you there!

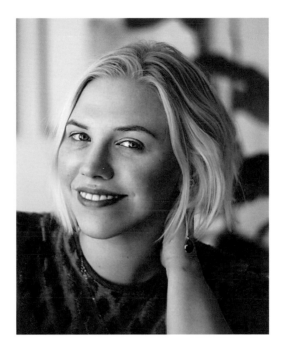

About the Author

Anuschka Rees is a writer from Berlin, where she lives with her books, cats, and boyfriend. Her first book *The Curated Closet* was a bestseller and has been translated into five languages.

🌐 anuschkarees.com

📷 anuschkarees

Also by Anuschka Rees:

The Curated Closet: A Simple System for Discovering Your Personal Style and Building Your Dream Wardrobe

The Curated Closet Workbook: Discover Your Personal Style and Build Your Dream Wardrobe

Acknowledgments

First of all, I need to thank the 606 women (plus a handful of men) who contributed their personal stories and thoughts for this book. Body image is such an intimate, loaded topic and I cannot overstate how much I appreciate your generosity, candor, vulnerability, wit, and insights.

I also want to thank the experts and professionals who shared their research and perspectives with me: Renee Engeln, PhD; Dr. Silja Vocks; Dr. Gail Dines; Evelyn Tribole, MS, RD; Ashton Applewhite; Caroline Dooner; Dr. Midge Wilson; Lexie Kite, PhD; Lindsay Kite, PhD; Dr. Roberto Olivardia; Emma Sanders; and Kelsey Miller. Your wisdom is the backbone of this book.

Kaitlin Ketchum, thank you for believing in this book, for understanding the big picture, and for making it happen. I could not have asked for a better partner for this book than you.

Lindsay Edgecombe, thank you for your guidance and your strength, and for always having my back.

To Marina Esmeraldo, Emma Campion, and Lisa Ferkel: Thank you for all of your hard work and a beautiful book design.

And thank you, Ben! For all of your love, calm optimism, and encouragement; for helping me organize my anxious writer's brain; and for endless evenings spent talking about body ideals, media messages, and hair removal practices. Thank you!

Bibliography

INTRODUCTION

The American Society for Aesthetic Plastic Surgery. "Cosmetic Surgery National Data Bank Statistics 2017." https://www.surgery.org/media/statistics.

National Eating Disorders Association, "Statistics & Research on Eating Disorders." https://www.nationaleating disorders.org/statistics-research-eating-disorders. Accessed February 2, 2018.

Phillips, Katharine A. *The Broken Mirror: Understanding and Treating Body Dysmorphic Disorder.* Oxford, UK: Oxford University Press, 1996.

Reba-Harreleson, Lauren, Ann Von Holle, Robert M. Hamer, Rebecca Swann, Mae Lynn Reyes, and Cynthia M. Bulik. "Patterns and Prevalence of Disordered Eating and Weight Control Behaviors in Women Ages 25—45." *Eating and Weight Disorders* 14, no. 4 (2009): e190—98.

Unilever. The Dove Global Beauty and Confidence Report, 2016. Accessed February 1, 2017.

BODY IMAGE 101

Ambrosini, Melissa. *Mastering Your Mean Girl: The No-BS Guide to Silencing Your Inner Critic and Becoming Wildly Wealthy, Fabulously Healthy, and Bursting with Love.* New York: TarcherPerigee, 2016.

Cash, Thomas F. *The Body Image Workbook: An Eight-Step Program for Learning to Like Your Looks.* Oakland, CA: New Harbinger Publications, Inc., 1997.

Dweck, Carol S. *Mindset: The New Psychology of Success.* New York: Random House, 2006.

Steinem, Gloria. *Revolution from Within: A Book of Self-Esteem.* Boston: Little, Brown and Company, 1993.

Thompson, Joel Kevin. "Body Image: Extent of Disturbance, Associated Features, Theoretical Models, Assessment Methodologies, Intervention Strategies, and a Proposal for a New DSM-IV Diagnostic Category-Body Image Disorder." *Progress in Behavior Modification* 28 (1992): 3—54.

Walker, D. C., and A. D. Murray. "Body Image Behaviors: Checking, Fixing, and Avoiding." In *Encyclopedia of Body Image and Human Appearance,* ed. Thomas F. Cash, 166—72. San Diego, CA: Elsevier Academic Press, 2012.

THE MEDIA

Engeln, Renee. *Beauty Sick: How the Cultural Obsession with Appearance Hurts Girls and Women.* New York: HarperCollins, 2017.

Graff, Kaitlin, Sarah Murnen, and Anna K. Krause. "Low-Cut Shirts and High-Heeled Shoes: Increased Sexualization across Time in Magazine Depictions of Girls." *Sex Roles* 69 (2013): 571—582.

Hatton, E., and M. N. Trautner. "Equal Opportunity Objectification? The Sexualization of Men and Women on the Cover of *Rolling Stone.*" *Sexuality & Culture* 15 (2011): 256.

Heldman, Caroline. "Sexual Objectification (Part 1): What Is It?" *The Society Pages,* July 12, 2012. https://thesocietypages.org/socimages/2012/07/02/sexual-objectification-part-1-what-is-it.

Kite, Lindsay. "Empowering or Objectifying: The Clashing Camps of Body Positivity." *Beauty Redefined*, January 5, 2016. https://beautyredefined.org/empowering-objectifying-body-positivity.

Kite, Lindsay, and Lexie Kite. "Stop Cheering for the Objectification of More Women." *Beauty Redefined*, January 12, 2017. https://beautyredefined.org/stop-cheering-objectification-of-more-women.

McKelle, Erin. "On Choice, Feminism, and Internalized Misogyny: Why We Participate in Patriarchal Oppression," *Everyday Feminism*. July 25, 2015. https://everydayfeminism.com/2014/07/choice-feminism-internalized-misogyny.

Rooney, Emma. "The Effects of Sexual Objectification on Women's Mental Health." *Online Publication of Undergraduate Studies* 7.2 (2016). 33—36.

Unilever. The Real Truth about Beauty Revisited: Dove Global Study 2010. Accessed February 1, 2017.

OTHER PEOPLE

Cash, Thomas F. *The Body Image Workbook: An Eight-Step Program for Learning to Like Your Looks.* Oakland, CA: New Harbinger Publications, Inc., 1997.

DeVoe, Jill Fleury, and Lynn Bauer. *Student Victimization in U.S. Schools: Results from the 2009 School Crime Supplement to the National Crime Victimization Survey* (NCES 2012-314). U.S. Department of Education, National Center for Education Statistics. Washington, DC: U.S. Government Printing Office, 2011.

Engeln, Renee, and Rachel H. Salk. "The Demographics of Fat Talk in Adult Women: Age, Body Size, and Ethnicity." *Journal of Health Psychology* 21, no. 8 (2016): 1655—64.

Hunger, Jeffrey M., and A. Janet Tomiyama. "Weight Labeling and Obesity. A 10-Year Longitudinal Study of Girls Aged 10—19." *JAMA Pediatrics* 168 (2014): 579—80.

Logel, Christine, Danu Anthony Stinson, Gregory R. Gunn, Joanne V. Wood, John G. Holmes, and Jessica J. Cameron. "A Little Acceptance Is Good for Your Health: Interpersonal Messages and Weight Change over time." *Personal Relationships* 21 (2014): 583—598.

Mills, Jacqueline, and Matthew Fuller-Tyszkiewicz. "Nature and Consequences of Positively Intended Fat Talk in Daily Life." *Body Image* 26 (2018): 38—49.

Musu-Gillette, Lauren, Anlan Zhang, Ke Wang, Jizhi Zhang, and Barbara A. Oudekerk. *Indicators of School Crime and Safety: 2016* (NCES 2017-064/NCJ 250650). National Center for Education Statistics, U.S. Department of Education, and Bureau of Justice Statistics, Office of Justice Programs, U.S. Department of Justice. Washington, DC. U.S. Government Printing Office, 2017.

National Eating Disorders Association. "Statistics & Research on Eating Disorders." https://www.nationaleatingdisorders.org/statistics-research-eating-disorders. Accessed June 20, 2018.

The Psychlopaedia Team (The Australian Psychological Society). "Why 'Fat Talk' Can Lead to Poor Body Image." *Psychlopaedia* (July 13, 2017). https://psychlopaedia.org/health/fat-talk-can-lead-poor-body-image.

Tomiyama, A. Janet. "Weight Stigma is Stressful: A Review of Evidence for the Cyclic Obesity/Weight-Based Stigma Model." *Appetite* 82 (2014): 8—15.

SELF-PERCEPTION

Bauer, A., et al. "Selective Visual Attention towards Oneself and Associated State Body Satisfaction: An Eye-Tracking Study in Adolescents with Different Types of Eating Disorders." *Journal of Abnormal Child Psychology* 45, no. 8 (November 2017): 1647—61.

Dove Real Beauty Sketches. "You're More Beautiful Than You Think." April 14, 2013. https://www.youtube.com/watch?v=litXW91UauE.

Grogan, Sarah. *Body Image: Understanding Body Dissatisfaction in Men, Women and Children.* London: Routledge, 2016.

Kite, Lindsay. "Not Picture Perfect? Bounce Back from a Body Image Blow." *Beauty Redefined*, May 19, 2017. https://beautyredefined.org/not-picture-perfect-bounce-back-from-a-body-image-blow.

McCabe, Marita P., Lina A. Ricciardelli, Geeta Sitaram, and Katherine Mikhail. "Accuracy of Body Size Estimation: Role of Biopsychosocial Variables." *Body Image* 3, no. 2 (2006): 163—73.

Mita, Theodore H., Marshall Dermer, and Jeffrey Knight. "Reversed Facial Images and the Mere-Exposure Hypothesis." *Journal of Personality and Social Psychology* 35 (1977): 597—601.

Nahman, Haley. "After 28 Years, I Still Don't Know What I Look Like." *Man Repeller*, October 18, 2017. https://www.manrepeller.com/2017/10/what-do-i-look-like.html.

Sincero, Jen. *You Are a Badass: How to Stop Doubting Your Greatness and Start Living an Awesome Life.* Philadelphia, PA: Running Press Adult, 2013.

Smeets, Elke, Anita Jansen, and Anne Roefs. "Bias for the (Un)Attractive Self: On the Role of Attention in Causing Body (Dis)Satisfaction." *Health Psychology* 30, no. 3 (2011): 360—67.

Thompson, Joel Kevin, and Richard Enrico Spana. "The Adjustable Light Beam Method for the Assessment of Size Estimation Accuracy: Description, Psychometrics and Normative Data." *International Journal of Eating Disorders* 7, no. 4 (1988): 521—26.

Voges, Mona, Claire-Marie Giabbiconi, Benjamine Schöne, Manuel Waldorf, Andrea S. Hartmann, and Silja Vocks. "Double Standards in Body Evaluation? The Influence of Identification with Body Stimuli on Ratings of Attractiveness, Body Fat, and Muscle Mass." *Eating and Weight Disorders: Studies on Anorexia, Bulimia and Obesity* (2017): 1—8. https://onlinelibrary.wiley.com/doi/pdf/10.1002/eat.22967

BEAUTY STANDARDS

Adams, Cecil, "Who Decided Women Should Shave Their Legs and Underarms?" *The Straight Dope,* February 6, 1991. http://www.straightdope.com/columns/read/625/who-decided-women-should-shave-their-legs-and-underarms.

Adichie, Chimamanda Ngozi. *Americanah.* New York: Alfred A. Knopf, 2013.

Applewhite, Ashton. *This Chair Rocks: A Manifesto against Ageism.* Networked Books, 2016.

Ashenburg, Katherine, "Why Do Americans Cherish Cleanliess? Look to War and Advertising." *New York Times*, updated May 28, 2013. https://www.nytimes.com/roomfordebate/2013/05/27/are-americans-too-obsessed-with-cleanliness/why-do-americans-cherish-cleanliess-look-to-war-and-advertising.

Bushak, Lecia. "History Of Body Image In America: How The 'Ideal' Female And Male Body Has Changed Over Time," *Medical Daily*. November 6, 2015. https://www.medicaldaily.com/history-body-image-america-how-ideal-female-and-male-body-has-changed-over-360492.

Byrd, Ayana, and Lori Tharps. *Hair Story: Untangling the Roots of Black Hair in America*. New York: St. Martin's Press, 2014.

Cash, Thomas F. *The Body Image Workbook: An Eight-Step Program for Learning to Like Your Looks*. Oakland, CA: New Harbinger Publications, Inc., 1997.

Chou, Jessica. "The Bizarre History of Body Hair." *Refinery 29*, May 8, 2015. http://www.refinery29.com/body-grooming-history.

Clinton, Hilary. *What Happened*. New York: Simon & Schuster, 2017.

Cooper, Helene. "Where Beauty Means Bleached Skin." *New York Times*, November 26, 2016. https://www.nytimes.com/2016/11/26/fashion/skin-bleaching-south-africa-women.html.

Davis, Kiri. "A Girl like Me." Video posted May 4, 2007. https://www.youtube.com/watch?v=YWyl77Yh1Gg.

Daycard, Laurène. "Cellulite Used to be Chill." *Vice*, April 7, 2016. https://broadly.vice.com/en_us/article/785g89/cellulite-used-to-be-chill.

Fisher, Carrie. Fisher quote from her personal twitter account @carrieffisher. December 29, 2015.

Hope, Christine. "Caucasian Female Body Hair and American Culture." *Journal of American Culture* 5 (1982): 93—99.

The International Society of Aesthetic Plastic Surgery. Global Aesthetic Survey, 2016. https://www.isaps.org/medical-professionals/isaps-global-statistics.

Johnson, Maisha Z. "Ten ways the beauty industry tells you being beautiful means being white," *Everyday Feminism*. January 3, 2016. https:/everydayfeminism.com/2016/01/when-beauty-equals-white.

Laan, Ellen, Daphne K. Martoredjo, Sara Hesselink, Nóinín Snijders, and Rik H. W. van Lunsen. "Young Women's Genital Self-Image and Effects of Exposure to Pictures of Natural Vulvas." *Journal of Psychosomatic Obstetrics & Gynecology* 38 (2016): 1—7.

Lawton, Georgina. "The Problems with the Natural Hair Movement." *Dazed*, May 9, 2016. http://www.dazeddigital.com/artsandculture/article/30536/1/the-problems-with-the-natural-hair-movement.

Lee, Michelle. "Lupita Nyong'o Opens Up about the Looks She and Her Hairstylist Created for *Allure's* March Issue." *Allure*, February 12, 2018. https://www.allure.com/story/lupita-nyongo-march-2018-cover-story-interview.

Lorena, Sammy. "The Psychology of Skin Whitening." *The Kolor Komplex*, January 21, 2017. https://www.kolorkomplex.com/kolorkomplex-culture/2017/1/5/the-psychology-of-skin-whitening.

Marshall, Sarah. "When, and Why, Did Women Start Dyeing Their Gray Hair?" *Elle*, September 18, 2015. https://www.elle.com/beauty/hair/news/a30556/when-and-why-did-women-start-dyeing-their-gray-hair.

Orenstein, Peggy. *Girls & Sex: Navigating the Complicated New Landscape.* New York: HarperCollins, 2016.

"Our Barbie Vaginas, Ourselves." *Mother Jones,* May/June 2016. http://www.motherjones.com/media/2016/05/our-waxed-barbie-vaginas-ourselves-1.

Patton, Tracey Owens. "Hey Girl, Am I More Than My Hair? African American Women and Their Struggles with Beauty, Body Image, and Hair." *NWSA Journal* 18, no. 2 (2006): 24–51.

Pierre-Louis, Kendra. "Beauty Standards Are Literally Toxic for Women of Color." *Popular Science,* August 16, 2017. https://www.popsci.com/personal-care-products-are-especially-toxic-for-women-color.

Rehman, Maliha. "Getting Rich from the Skin Lightening Trade." *Business of Fashion.* September 27, 2017. https://www.businessoffashion.com/articles/global-currents/profiting-from-the-skin-lightening-trade.

Rowen, Tami S., Thomas W. Gaither, Mohannad Awad, Charles Osterberg, Alan W. Shindel, and Benjamin N. Breyer. "Pubic Hair Grooming Prevalence and Motivation among Women in the United States." *JAMA Dermatology* 152, no. 10 (2016): 1106–13.

Russell-Cole, Kathy, Midge Wilson, and Ronald E. Hall. *The Color Complex: The Politics of Skin Color in a New Millennium.* New York: Anchor Books, 2013.

Scherker, Amanda. "7 Ways the Beauty Industry Convinced Women That They Weren't Good Enough." *Huffington Post,* updated December 6, 2017. https://www.huffingtonpost.com/2014/04/29/beauty-industry—women_n_5127078.html.

Sutton, Denise H. *Globalizing Ideal Beauty: Women, Advertising, and the Power of Marketing.* Basingstoke, UK: Palgrave Macmillan US, 2009.

Thompson, Cheryl. "Black Women and Identity: What's Hair Got to Do with It?" *Politics and Performativity,* 22, no. 1: 2008-2009.

Vox. "Why the Market for Skin Whitening Is Growing." Video posted January 4, 2018. https://www.youtube.com/watch?v=Cjzvvgmg1NU.

Wolf, Naomi. *The Beauty Myth: How Images of Beauty Are Used against Women.* London: Vintage, 1991.

MORE THAN A BODY

Cash, Thomas F. *The Body Image Workbook: An Eight-Step Program for Learning to Like Your Looks.* Oakland, CA: New Harbinger Publications, Inc., 1997.

Fennel, Melanie. *Overcoming Low Self-Esteem: A Self-Help Guide Using Cognitive Behavioural Techniques,* 2nd ed. London: Hatchett UK, 2016.

I CAN'T TONIGHT, I FEEL FAT

Cash, Thomas F. *The Body Image Workbook: An Eight-Step Program for Learning to Like Your Looks.* Oakland, CA: New Harbinger Publications, Inc., 1997.

SOCIAL MEDIA

Engeln, Renee. *Beauty Sick: How the Cultural Obsession with Appearance Hurts Girls and Women.* New York: HarperCollins, 2017.

Halliwell, Emma, Alice Easun, and Diana Harcourt. "Body Dissatisfaction: Can a Short Media Literacy Message Reduce Negative Media Exposure Effects amongst Adolescent Girls?" *British Journal of Health Psychology* 16 (2011): 396–403.

Kite, Lindsay, and Lexie Kite. "Selfies and Self-Objectification: A Not-So-Pretty Picture." *Beauty Redefined*, March 13, 2014, https://beautyredefined.org/selfies-and-objectification.

Simmons, Rachel. "How Social Media Is a Toxic Mirror." *Time*, August 19, 2016. http://time.com/4459153/social-media-body-image.

FOOD & FITNESS

Boepple, Leah, and J. Kevin Thompson. "A Content Analytic Comparison of Fitspiration and Thinspiration Websites." *International Journal of Eating Disorders* 49, no. 1 (January 2016): 98–101.

Dooner, Caroline. *The F*ck It Diet: Stop Dieting and Start Taking Up Space.* New York: HarperCollins, 2019.

Intuitive Eating Studies. "Creating a Healthy Relationship with Food, Mind & Body." http://www.intuitiveeating.org/resources/studies.

Kalm, Leah M., and Richard D. Semba. "They Starved So That Others Be Better Fed: Remembering Ancel Keys and The Minnesota Experiment." *Journal of Nutrition* 135, no. 6 (June 2005): 1347–52.

Kite, Lindsay, and Lexie Kite. "Your Body Is Powerful. Use It as an Instrument, Not an Ornament." *Beauty Redefined*. December 18, 2014. https://beautyredefined.org/body-is-instrument-not-ornament.

Spinardi, Josie. *How to Have Your Cake and Your Skinny Jeans Too: Stop Binge Eating, Overeating and Dieting for Good Get the Naturally Thin Body You Crave from the Inside Out.* Walnut Creek, CA: Twirl Media, 2014.

Tribole, Evelyn, and Elyse Resch. *Intuitive Eating: A Revolutionary Program That Works.* New York: St. Martin's Press/Griffin Publishing, 2012.

BEAUTY ROUTINES

Fey, Tina. *Bossypants.* Boston: Little, Brown, 2013.

COSMETIC SURGERY

Honigman, Roberta, Katharine A. Phillips, and David J. Castle. "A Review of Psychosocial Outcomes for Patients Seeking Cosmetic Surgery." *Plastic and Reconstructive Surgery* 113, no. 4 (2004): 1229–37.

Von Soest, Tilmann, Ingela Lundin Kvalem, Helge Einar Roald, and Knut C. Skolleborg. "The Effects of Cosmetic Surgery on Body Image, Self-Esteem, and Psychological Problems." *Journal of Plastic, Reconstructive & Aesthetic Surgery* 62, no. 10 (2009): 1238–44.

Index

C

D

E

F

Food, relationship with, 144–45, 147.
See also Eating

G

Gibson, Dana Charles, 82
Gibson girl, 82
A Girl Like Me, 102–3
Grooming standards
    effects of, 97
    as hygiene issue, 96, 98–99
    recent, 91, 93

H

Hair
    African-American women and, 103–5
    gray, 94–95
    leg, 94, 96, 99
    pubic, 100, 102
    underarm, 94, 98–99
Hall, Ronald, 103, 106
Harper's Bazaar, 98, 99
Help, seeking professional, 9

I

Inner voice
    negative, 32–35, 121, 123–24
    positive, 117
Instagram. *See* Social media
Intuitive eating, 146, 149

J

Judgment, fear of, 121, 123–24

K

Kite, Lexie, 47, 133
Kite, Lindsay, 42, 47, 133

L

Labiaplasty, 88–89
Ladder of success, 127–28
Lawton, Georgina, 104
Leg hair, 94, 96, 99

M

Media
    beauty standards and, 1–2, 36–37, 39–40
    empowering messages in, 36
    literacy, 130
    See also Social media
Mills, Jacqueline, 62
Mirrors
    avoiding, 128
    reality and, 71–74
Modeling, 49–50
Models, plus-size, 84
Moss, Kate, 83

Published in the United States by Ten Speed Press, an imprint of the Crown
Publishing Group, a division of Penguin Random House LLC, New York.
www.crownpublishing.com
www.tenspeed.com

Ten Speed Press and the Ten Speed Press colophon are registered
trademarks of Penguin Random House LLC.

Library of Congress Cataloging-in-Publication Data
Names: Rees, Anuschka, author.
Title: Beyond beautiful : a practical guide to being happy, confident, and
    you in a looks-obsessed world / Anuschka Rees.
Description: Callifornia : Ten Speed Press, 2019. | Includes bibliographical
    references and index.
Identifiers: LCCN 2018045371
Subjects: LCSH: Self-actualization (Psychology) | Clothing and dress. |
    Beauty, Personal. | BISAC: SELF-HELP / Personal Growth / Happiness. |
    HEALTH & FITNESS / Beauty & Grooming.
Classification: LCC BF637.S4 R447 2019 | DDC 158.1—dc23
LC record available at https://lccn.loc.gov/2018045371

Hardcover ISBN: 978-0-399-58209-7
eBook ISBN: 978-0-399-58210-3

Printed in China

Design by Lisa Ferkel

10 9 8 7 6 5 4 3 2 1

First Edition